Health Beyond Medicine

Some Reflections on the Politics and Sociology of Health in India

Vikas Bajpai
Anoop Saraya

AAKAR

Health Beyond Medicine: Some Reflections on the Politics and Sociology of Health in India
Vikas Bajpai and Anoop Saraya

First Published 2018

ISBN 978-93-5002-527-7

Published by
AAKAR BOOKS
28 E Pocket IV, Mayur Vihar Phase I
Delhi 110 091 India
aakarbooks@gmail.com

Laser Typeset at
Arpit Printographers, Delhi 110 032

Printed at
Sapra Brothers, Delhi 110 092

Contents

Foreword

There are broadly two kinds of medical practitioners: those who regard treating patients day in and day out as their primary goal and those who, besides being good medical practitioners, also take time off treating patients to reflect on the social, economic and political environment within which they work and how it impacts on provisioning of health care. The authors belong to this latter category. They have tried in this book to look at health care policies and practices and to assess their consequences for the development of a health care framework for the country keeping in view the enormous social cultural and economic diversity of the country in mind. Of special interest is their concern for the poor and disadvantaged sections of society when it comes to access to health care. As they put it, 'A large section of the middle classes and the intelligentsia, among them medical professionals included, do get allured by . . . assurances and promises. Apart from being the result of their class position, such responses are also conditioned by the overt and covert training that the system itself imparts to these sections of society. They get used to analytical frameworks which rationalize the situation as it is rather than question the injustices inherent in it.'

The authors take as their starting point the recommendations of the Bhore Committee which was the first attempt to take stock of future provisioning of health care in Independent India. The heart of the Committee was in the right place. It did not look at the future of provisioning of health care in isolation. Instead, it took a comprehensive view of health care in the larger context of the social and political economy of the country. It recognized that for a country as large and as diverse as India and marked by social and economic inequities required that an integrated approach was not only necessary but also imperative. It categorically stated that in a democratic country witnessing a revolution of rising expectations the responsibility for providing health to citizens must fall on the State.

The final outcome of the deliberations of the Committee was far from sufficient and satisfactory. For one thing, the Committee came out with what may be called a system's approach to health care looking at health in terms of diagnostic and curative health care as the cornerstone of health policies. Second, it pushed a welfarist approach to health care rather than advocating a right's approach for securing health for the teeming millions the majority of whom were poor and eked out a pitiable existence. The difference between the two approaches is significant. In one the poor and the disadvantages are treated as recipients of health care from a benign government. In the other they are vested with a positive entitlement to health care. Perhaps, some of these lacunae arose from the fundamental reality of rising expectations, the alliance between the British ruling classes and the Indian political leadership, continuance of the colonial paradigm of governance, and the great chasm between a limited elite and the vast majority of Indians living in the rural areas and urban slums.

The deficiencies and weaknesses of the health care system in the country are too well known to need detailed recounting here. Several features of the health care system as it exists are worth noting. Public health expenditure remains very low in India. Less than 1 per cent of the GDP is spent on public health care services in India. Even though real state expenditure on health has increased by 7 per cent annually in recent years, central government expenditure has plateaued. Economically weaker states are particularly susceptible to low public health investment. Many state governments also fail to use allocated funds, but this might simply reflect structural weaknesses in the system and that need to be addressed with more resources and a different approach to provision and delivery of health care. It remains to be seen if the flow of greater share of the central taxes under the 14th finance commission recommendations will increase investment in health.

There is a large gap in the health care system between urban and rural areas. The inequity among regions is due to a lack of health care resources and infrastructure in the rural region. Compounding the issue, most of the population resides in rural part of the country (68.84 per cent). Consequently, only a quarter of the Indian population has access to allopathic medicine, and most of them live in urban areas. The majority of the hospitals are privately owned and located in cities due to the sector's awareness of the health-related issues and financial viability. However, the disadvantaged urban population cannot afford the private facilities in the cities. In response to this lack of availability, the Indian government has launched the National Urban Health Mission. Its principal mission is to ensure adequate resources and to reduce health problems for the vulnerable poor urban sector. Under this mission, the government pays the insurance premium for select individuals and works in conjunction with the private sector. While the National Urban Health Mission has had some success, it does not address India's biggest health care concern. The rural regions have less access to modern medical treatments and depend more on traditional treatment such as unani and acupuncture. The rural population has significantly less financial capital and relies heavily on government funded medical facilities.

There is also a great disparity in the distribution of health care facilities between regions and states. For instance, there is one government hospital bed for every 614 people in Goa compared with one every 8,789 people in Bihar. The care provided in these facilities is also not up to the mark. For example, in 2011, six out of every 10 hospitals in the less developed states did not provide intensive care. The National Rural Health Mission was launched by the Government of India with the goal to provide effective health care to rural people with a focus on 18 states which had poor public health indicators and/or weak infrastructure. However, even this bold initiative has had limited impact. Only 2 per cent of doctors are in rural areas where 68 per cent of the population lives. Non-availability of diagnostic tools and increasing reluctance of qualified and experienced health care professionals to practice in rural, under-equipped and financially less lucrative rural areas remains a big challenge. Rural medical practitioners are highly sought after by residents of rural areas as they are more financially affordable and geographically accessible than practitioners working in the formal public health care sector. There have also been reports of kickbacks for referrals, irrational drug prescribing and unnecessary interventions.

The World Health Organization's 2000 global health care profile ranked India's health care system 112th out of 190 countries. This survey highlighted four major health concerns for India that still are prominent today. The first concern is the high vulnerability of young children. Among children under five, 43.5 per cent are underweight (the highest percentage in the world) and 6.6 per cent die before their fifth birthday. Analysis of National Family Health Survey Data for 2005-06 (the most recent available dataset for analysis) showed the under-five mortality rate for the poorest quartile eight states. The highest under-five mortality rate in the poorest quartile occurred in Uttar Pradesh (110 per 1,000 live births), India's most populous state, which had 44.4 million urban dwellers in the 2011 census followed by Rajasthan (102), Madhya Pradesh (98), Jharkhand (90) Bihar (85), Delhi (74), and Maharashtra (50). The sample for West Bengal was too small for analysis of under-five mortality rate. In Uttar Pradesh the rate was four times that of the rest of the urban populations in Maharashtra and Madhya Pradesh. In Madhya Pradesh, the under-five mortality rate among its poorest quartile was more than three times that of the rest of its urban population.

Likewise, among India's urban population, one should note the much lower proportion of mothers receiving maternity care among the poorest quartile; only 54 per cent of pregnant women had at least three ante-natal care visits compared to 83 per cent for the rest of the urban population. Less than a quarter of mothers within the poorest quartile received adequate maternity care in Bihar (12 per cent), and Uttar Pradesh (20 per cent), and less than half in Madhya Pradesh (38 per cent), Delhi (41 per cent), Rajasthan (42 per cent), and Jharkhand (48 per cent). Availing three or more ante-natal check-ups during pregnancy among the poorest quartile was better in West Bengal (71 per cent) and Maharashtra (73 per cent).

For India's urban population in 2005–06, 54 per cent of children were stunted, and 47 per cent underweight in the poorest urban quartile, compared to 33 per cent and 26 per cent, respectively, for the rest of the urban population. Children under five years being stunted was particularly high among the poorest quartile of the urban populations in Uttar Pradesh (64 per cent), Maharashtra (63 per cent), Bihar (58 per cent), Delhi (58 per cent), Madhya Pradesh (55 per cent), Rajasthan (53 per cent), and slightly better in Jharkhand (49 per cent). Even in the better-performing states close to half of the children under-five were stunted among the poorest quartile, being 48 per cent in West Bengal. High levels of stunted growth and being under-weight for age among the urban poor in India points to repeated infections, depleting the child's nutritional reserves, owing to sub-optimal physical environment. It is also indicative of high levels of food insecurity among this segment of the population. A study carried out in the slums of Delhi showed that 51 per cent of slum families were food insecure.

There is a growing chasm between public and private health care. According to National Family Health Survey-3, the private medical sector remains the primary source of health care for 70 per cent of households in urban areas and 63 per cent of households in rural areas. Reliance on public and private health care sector varies significantly between states. Several reasons are cited for relying on private rather than public sector; the main reason at the national level is poor quality of care in the public sector, with more than 57 per cent of households pointing to this as the reason for a preference for private health care. Most of the public health care caters to the rural areas; and the poor quality arises from the reluctance of experienced health care providers to visit the rural areas. Consequently, the majority of the public health care system catering to the rural and remote areas relies on inexperienced and unmotivated interns who are mandated to spend time in public health care clinics as part of their curricular requirement. Other major reasons are distance of the public sector facility, long wait times, and inconvenient hours of operation. The study conducted by IMS Institute for Healthcare Informatics in 2013 across 12 states in over 14,000 households indicated a steady increase in the usage of private health care facilities over the last 25 years for both Out Patient and In Patient services, across rural and urban areas.

With the help of numerous government subsidies in the 1980s, private health providers entered the market. Opening up of the market in the 90s gave further impetus to the development of the private health sector in India. Most of the health care capacity added after 2005 has been in the private sector, or in partnership with the private sector. Private health care providers in India typically offer high quality treatment at highly unreasonable costs as there is no regulatory authority or statutory neutral body to check for medical malpractices. On 27 May 2012, the popular actor Aamir Khan's programme *Satyamev Jayate* did an episode on "Does Healthcare Need Healing?" which highlighted the high costs and other malpractices adopted by private clinics and hospitals.

Given the quality of care available, few frequent public sector hospitals. The National Sample Survey Office (NSSO) numbers show a decrease in the use of public hospitals over the past two decades—only 32 per cent of urban Indians use them now, compared with 43 per eent in 1995-96. However, a significant portion of these private practitioners may not be qualified or are under-qualified. For instance, a study in rural Madhya Pradesh found that only 11 per cent of the sampled health care providers had a medical degree, and only 53 per cent had completed high school. Moreover, the many new institutions set up in the past decade, encouraged by commercial incentives, have often fuelled corrupt practices and failed to offer quality health education.

Overall, the governance and accountability has been remarkably weak in the health care system in India. In the past 5 years, the government has introduced several new laws to strengthen governance of the health system, but many of these laws have not been widely implemented. In some instances, the scope of regulations is still unclear, and there are fears that these laws have hindered public health trials led by non-commercial entities. Thus, inadequate public investment in health, the missing trust and engagement between various health care sectors and poor coordination between state and central governments are the main constraints why universal health care is not assured in India. At the heart of these constraints is the apparent unwillingness on the part of the state to prioritize health as a fundamental public good, central to India's developmental aspirations, on par with education. Put simply, there is no clear ownership of the idea of universal health coverage within the government.

The authors make a strong case for a reorientation of the architecture of health care in India and indicate the directions along which we must move to ensure universal health care. For one thing, there is need to place health care within the overall frame of the structure of Indian society and the balance of forces that shape the prospects for a change in the health care policies. As they put it, 'Caste, class, gender, religion and ethnicity are important determinants of health outcomes among the people which no health service system can ignore. The question . . . is not whether health services and health personnel discriminate between people on the basis of these affiliations, but to what extent are they aware of the impact of these factors on the health of the people ... ? Inability to adequately appraise these factors leads to a victim blaming approach where the suffering people are held to be their own enemies.'

The book promises to be refreshing reading not only for health professionals and policy makers but also for general readers who are bothered about the state of health care in India.

New Delhi **Imtiaz Ahmad**

Authors' Note

At long last we are happy that this volume is finally being put out for your scrutiny. The title of the book—*Health Beyond Medicine: Some Reflections on the Politics and Sociology of Health in India* itself encapsulates an introduction to its contents. But before we dwell on the contents, a few words regarding why we felt the need for this book would be helpful in putting things in perspective.

It is well acknowledged, at least amongst health activists, academics and large sections of the policy establishment, that health is a socially produced phenomenon. There is a huge body of literature available to testify to the role of the 'social determinants of health.' But all of this notwithstanding, when it comes to planning for health, the entrenched wisdom among the people who matter privileges health care services, and among them also the provisioning of curative care services as an expedient to ensuring people's health. Furthermore, an impression is sought to be created that the health services themselves, and the nature and process of their development, if not immune to social, economic and political influences, is at least undertaken by the ruling elite in a manner as to objectively serve the best interest of the people. It is portrayed that the system is aware of the plight of the socially and economically marginalized people and does try to build safeguards for them. The imperfections that are still left shall be remedied with further progress of the country.

A large section of the middle classes and the intelligentsia, among them medical professionals included, do get allured by such assurances and promises. Apart from being the result of their class position, such responses are also conditioned by the overt and covert training that the system itself imparts to these sections of the society. They get used to analytical frameworks which rationalize the situation as it is rather than question the injustices inherent in it. Well meaning people at large and amongst them those who can make a difference to the development of a pro-people health system, such as the health professionals and workers, start conceptualizing health problems and their possible solutions from the perspective of those who monopolize these services rather than seeing them from the perspective of the impoverished majority, thereby making the correctives that much more difficult to implement.

Nevertheless, like so many other evils of Indian democracy, the unpalatable realities of the health services system in the country, the miseries of our suffering people and their aspirations for a better future, have an uncanny way of ripping open the inconsistencies in the rosy picture sought to be painted before us, thereby posing a *disconcerting dilemma* for many amongst us who are relatively better off in the system; may even be benefiting from it, and yet wish to partake in the trials and travails of those seventy-seven per cent of Indians who, as the report of the National Commission on Employment in the Unorganized Sector (NCEUS) told us, subsisted on less than twenty rupees a day, at least in 2007. It may also be noted that as per the same report it took a daily per capita expenditure of mere ninety-three rupees to be counted as a rich Indian.

This book is an attempt to cash in on the *'window of opportunity'* offered by this *'disconcerting dilemma'* in order to make a difference to the health of the hundreds of millions of impoverished Indians. The book attempts to remove the analytical blinkers put on our minds by the ruling elite such that we can see clearly the links between the social, economic and political structure of our society, the shape of our health services system and the health of the people.

India's health services system is one of the most privatized and iniquitous in the world with the share of public spending on health being one of the lowest. Despite many of its acclaimed successes, which by no means are unique to India with many of the less developed countries having achieved much more than us, the fact remains that health care has increasingly become a commodity access to which is conditioned by the purchasing power of the people. And if the overall purchasing power to fulfil all sorts of physical needs necessary for human sustenance is just rupees twenty a day, one can imagine the quality of health care that is accessible to the poor in India. Despite this, a change still appears nowhere on the horizon.

The first step towards bringing about change is to see and understand the reality for what it is. The first few chapters of the book take us through the history of the development of the health services in India, beginning with the recommendations of the landmark report of the Bhore Committee that laid the foundations of the public health services in independent India. The contradictions between the developed and the developing countries and the class contradictions within the Indian society has been the key heuristic device for interpreting the history of health services in independent India including the present state of affairs and the proposed strategy for future development. Even as we invite you to form your own opinion on the subject, our analysis shows that little, if any, of the maladies in the health services system of India is inadvertent; the development of the system has been exactly as the ruling classes have wanted it to be.

The most important implication of this is that we need to take far greater interest in changing the current balance of forces in the Indian society which impacts most heavily on the development policy making rather than be satisfied with taking one blind hit after another by tweaking the limited set of policy instruments that are generally acceptable under the present dispensation.

Caste, class, gender, religion and ethnicity are important determinants of health outcomes amongst the people which no health services system can afford to ignore. The question here is not whether health services and health personnel discriminate between the people on the basis of these affiliations, but to what extent are they aware of the impact of these factors on the health of the people and how do they account for these? Inability to adequately appraise these factors leads to a victim blaming approach where the suffering people are held to be their own enemies. The worries that are often expressed on account of the burgeoning population of the poor are actually a part of this victim blaming. We have attempted to take a closer look at these factors in some of the chapters.

It is important to acknowledge here that this is not the first book of its kind and indeed there shall always be scope for many more books dealing with these issues till such time that a qualitative shift for better comes about. We hope that this book shall succeed in taking the conceptualization of health amongst its readers firmly beyond health care alone and integrate it with the larger societal conditions.

Your critical opinion would be appreciated.

Vikas Bajpai
(drvikasbajpai@gmail.com)

Anoop Saraya
(ansaraya@yahoo.com)

1

A Social, Political, and Public Health: Analysis of the Bhore Committee Recommendations*

Introduction

Even as the move for transfer of power from the British to the nationalist leaders of India was afoot, the then British government of India was faced with the challenge of setting up the framework of governance for the various functions the new independent Indian state would have to perform when it came into being; provision of health care was one such important function. Needless to say, the challenges confronting India in terms of improving the condition of health of her people were quite overwhelming, to say the least, with minimal infrastructure to tackle the gargantuan task at hand. Under the circumstances, the Government of India set up a Health Survey and Development Committee in 1943, popularly known as the Bhore Committee, deriving its name from that of its chairman, Sir Joseph Bhore. The Committee was charged with the task of undertaking:

1. A broad survey of the present position in regard to health conditions and health organization in British India; and
2. Recommendations for future developments.

The Committee finally submitted its report in 1946 in four volumes.

---

* This chapter had earlier been published in the journal *Social Change*, Vol. 41 (2): 215-231 in the year 2011 in a slightly modified form. It is being reproduced here with permission from the journal.

It suggested a short-term plan to be achieved over a period of 10 years and a long-term plan to be put in place over a period of 40 years to develop India's health services.

Although even today India has failed to fully achieve even the objectives of the short-term plan, yet the very idea of the Bhore Committee remains the most enduring image in the struggle for the development of health services in India because of the breadth and comprehensiveness of the Committee's vision. The recommendations of the Committee are remarkably prescient, far-reaching and all-encompassing. The present disarray in the Indian health services system makes them appear even more so. Just as the Beveridge Committee's recommendations led to the formation of the National Health Service (NHS) in the UK (Abel-Smith, 1992), so the Bhore Committee recommendations set out a blueprint for the development of the health services system in India. The difference is that while in the UK all, from Queen to pauper, seek the services of the NHS, in India we have accomplished a surgical division between costly private health care for the rich and a poor public health care service for the poor.

The Bhore Committee was not without a specific historical and political context. Its recommendations came against the background of the world capitalism's greatest crisis of the 20th century, the Second World War, which heralded the emergence of the Soviet Union as a new superpower along with virtually half of Europe turning red and the Communist movement in Asia gaining ground in China. In India too there was a great resurgence of both nationalist and left movements.

All these developments created reverberations in the hearts and minds of the working people of the West and also the oppressed people of the colonized countries, forcing their governments to take cognisance of the rising social and economic aspirations of their people. Besides this, there was also a fear that the rising tide of Communism would sweep India into its fold.

The Beveridge Committee in the UK identified five great social evils: squalor, ignorance, want, idleness, and disease that needed to be dealt with on priority. In conjunction with the Keynesian model of economic development, it heralded the emergence of a 'welfare state' in the UK, while the leaders of the Indian National

Congress in India modelled themselves as the messiahs of socialism in the subcontinent. There was a considerable confluence of interest between the British ruling classes and the leaders of the Indian National Congress, which in 1928 had demanded merely 'dominion status' under the British Crown (P.N. Chopra et al., 2005). The British, for their part, were keen to keep India within the British Commonwealth (Singh, 1985) and motivating an urge to assist the Congress leadership.

It has been widely argued that what happened in 1947 was a mere transfer of power from the British to Indian hands with little if any change in the structure of the Indian state or any radical redistribution of resources in the society. Even the constitutional and the legal arrangement that was to guide the scheme of things in 'independent India' was virtually retained as had been under British rule, with several sections of the 'Government of India Act' of 1935 being reproduced verbatim in the Indian Constitution (Indian Courts, 2009; Pylee, 2002). Most importantly, the colonial construct of the defence forces (globalsecurity.org, 2010) and the police was retained as such (Das and Varma, 1998).

Continuance of the colonial paradigm implies not just the continuance of the formal structure of governance, but also its attitude towards the people.

This background of the conditions obtaining in the period when the Bhore Committee was constituted gives us an idea of the kind of influences that shaped the recommendations of the Committee. The rising aspirations of the people, the collaboration between the British ruling classes and the Indian leadership, and the continuance of the colonial governance paradigm all helped to shape the Committee's recommendations.

The Positive Aspects of the Committee's Recommendations

It will be appropriate to begin by acknowledging the most positive contributions of the Committee, and it is in these that we find an acknowledgement of the rising aspirations of the people of India from the government of a country that was about to gain independence after 200 years of colonial rule. The British were conscious of these and it was in their political and economic interests to lay a framework that would assist the Indian leadership to address these aspirations.

Foregrounding the Role of the State in the Provision of Health

It is here that the ideological trends in the international and the national politics of the time seem to have most impacted the Committee. In the post-Second World War scenario, the state had begun to occupy a position of pre-eminence across countries in the developed world. The Committee very consciously did not make the emerging Indian Republic an exception to this trend and argued for free 'universal health care' to be provided by the state. It stated:

> The idea that the state should assume full responsibility for all measures, curative and preventive, which are necessary for safeguarding the health of the nation, is developing as a logical sequence. The modern trend is towards the provision of as complete a health service as possible by the state and the inclusion, within its scope, of the largest possible proportion of the community. The need for assuring the distribution of medical benefits to all, irrespective of their ability to pay, has also received recognition (Government of India, 1946, Vol. II, pp. 7, 12).

Giving primacy to the needs of India's poor, in the plan to build the health services, the Committee proposed entirely free health services (Ibid., Vol. II, p. 14) to be provided by a full-time cadre of salaried government doctors as against private practitioners (Ibid., Vol. II, pp. 14-15).

Foregrounding Health in the Policy Framework

Emphasizing the need for the 'health programme' to be given 'high priority' in the allocation of available resources, the Committee said:

> We feel we can safely assert that a nation's wealth, prosperity and advancement, whether in the economic or the intellectual sphere, are conditioned by the state of its physical well-being...
>
> ... We need no further justification for attempting to evolve a comprehensive plan which must inevitably cover a very wide field and necessarily entail large expenditure, if it is to take into account all the more important factors which go to the building up of a healthy, virile and dynamic people (Ibid., Vol. II, p. 2).

The report went on to state:

> To shut our eyes to the consequences which a halting, ineffective and

> timid health policy imposes on the country can only result in perpetuating a tragedy which is as poignant on the national as on the individual side.

Little would the Committee have imagined that the entire experience of governance post-1947 would so catastrophically bear out their prophecy. Going by the way 'Health' has been treated in the state policy post-1947, elevates these quotations way above good semantics.

An Epidemiological Approach to Public Health Diagnosis and Planning

That the report is a very well written document is recognized. However, its salience lies in the epidemiological method adopted in diagnosing the real issues confronting India in the health arena. The Committee through its deliberations collated a huge amount of data on the topics below, to diagnose what ailed India's millions and drew up priorities for action. The areas that came under the Committee's scrutiny were (Ibid., Vol. I):

- Data on health infrastructure available in India, the number of medical and paramedical health personnel available, the adequacy of their training, the types of organizations involved in providing medical relief, the nature of services provided by them, and the conditions of service of the various health personnel.
- The status of availability of various therapeutic substances, instruments, and appliances, and the facilities for their production and the control of trade in these substances and equipment.
- Detailed data on the nutritional status of the people in various parts of India, data on production of food grains and animal products, and the institutional mechanisms for control of adulteration of food, supervision of the production and sale of food in public, and an analysis of food storage and distribution.
- The Committee undertook an in-depth analysis on the health services for vulnerable groups such as mothers and children and the schoolchildren.

- Great care and consideration was given to the poor standards of health of India's workforce; a section which seems to have gone beyond the pale of health policy in independent India.
- A separate chapter was devoted to an in-depth analysis of morbidity and mortality due to diseases that posed the greatest public health hazards in India and listed the facilities available to deal with these problems.

We may well say, 'well isn't this the obvious way to go about it; what is so great?' To absorb the full import of the Committee's methodology, one need only compare it with the profound absence of this approach in health policy even after so many years of independence and the acclaimed advances in knowledge, institutional mechanisms, and technological capabilities of the Indian state. Compared to the thoroughness of the epidemiological approach of the Bhore Committee, the 'Mission Document' of the National Rural Health Mission (NRHM) is no more than a bullet point presentation that does not even attempt to analyse the reasons for the dismal state of health in rural India (Government of India, 2005). In the words of Dr D. Banerji, NRHM is nothing more than a celebration of 'public health quackery' (Banerji, 2005).

A Systems Approach to Public Heath

The terms of reference of the Committee constrained the scope of its enquiry to 'review primarily those activities which can reasonably be regarded as falling within the scope of health administration' (Government of India, 1946, Vol. I, p. 4). However, this failed to obscure in any way the importance of health as a multidimensional phenomenon in the deliberations of the Committee. Throughout the text of its report the Committee adopted a 'health systems view' of health problems in India rather than confining itself within the narrow confines of 'health services system'.

The Committee said:

> While recognizing that it is not within the scope of our enquiry to suggest ways and means by which poverty and unemployment should be eliminated, we feel that our survey of the causes of ill-

> health in India will not be complete without drawing attention to the profound influence that these factors exert on the health of the community. In a reaffirmation of the principles regarding the health policy in connection with discussions on the Beveridge Report, the British Medical Association emphasized that 'the health of the people depends primarily upon the social and environmental conditions under which they live and work, upon security against fear and want, upon nutritional standards, upon educational facilities, and upon the facilities for exercise and leisure' (Ibid., Vol. I, p. 17).

It is illuminating to compare this comment with the mention of 'poverty' in the NRHM Mission Document: 'Over 25% of hospitalized Indians fall below the poverty line because of hospital expenses' and 'improved hospital care subsidized under the Janani Suraksha Yojana (JSY) for the Below Poverty Line families'. There is no third mention of the word 'poverty' and mention of 'unemployment' simply does not occur in the document (Government of India, 2005): lest the mandarins of 'Nirman Bhawan' (the building where the 'Ministry of Health and Family Welfare' is located) fret about something as irrelevant as the relationship between 'unemployment' and health.

It is not just the mention of 'poverty' that testifies to the 'systemic' approach of the Committee; they go on to state unambiguously:

> The modern public health movement is not concerned solely with the prevention of disease. It has the broader aim of creating an environment in which each individual can develop his potential fully and completely (Government of India, 1946, Vol. II, p. 69).

The Committee fully endorsed the statement of the 'Nutrition Committee' that:

> The general raising of the dietary standards throughout the country is an economic problem, the solution of which is dependent on the scientific development of agriculture. animal husbandry and fisheries, and the simultaneous development of industrial resources.... Agriculture and economic policy must be established which have as their primary objective the betterment of diet. A food policy is necessary, and this must be firmly based en nutritional science (Ibid., Vol. II, pp. 70-1).

This is in sharp contrast to the pedantic debate on the Food Security

Bill in the deliberations of the National Advisory Council, as if food security is just a matter of deciding whether to give 35 kg or 25 kg of food grains to below poverty line families or whether or not to make the public distribution system universal (*The Hindu*, 2010).

The Committee included in separate chapters its recommendations on important issues from the public health point of view on 'Environmental Hygiene', 'Rural and Urban Housing', 'Town and Village Planning', 'Public Health Engineering', 'Professional Education', 'Medical Research', etc. (Government of India, 1946, Vol. II, pp. 70-1). It is indeed remarkable that such an important programme as the NRHM makes no reference of the need to create institutional mechanisms to meet the demand of training huge numbers of public health professionals with social, political, and epidemiological competence that such a programme essentially requires. The only mention is that of training Accredited Social Health Activists (ASHAs) (Government of India, 2005) and that too has now been outsourced to NGOs.

Concept of Integrated and Universal Health care

Universal access to integrated (preventive, promotive, and rehabilitative) health care to this day remains the cherished public health goal. The Committee firmly rooted its proposals for the long and the short-term plans in complete accordance with these lofty public health ideals. It said:

> We consider that a combination of curative and preventive health work is in the best interests of the community and of the professional efficiency of the medical staff employed. In fact the two functions cannot be separated without detriment to the health of the community (Government of India, 1946, Vol. II, p. 40).

We need only compare this notion of integrated health care with the enormous dichotomy between the preventive care for rural India and concentration of curative care in urban India that has been the outcome of the development of health services in 'Independent' India. Perhaps some of the greatest ideas are also the simplest; that however does not always ensure that they are put into practice as simply.

There is an erroneous impression in the minds of some scholars that in its proposed short-term programme the Committee proposed coverage of only a fifth of the population in the initial five years and barely half the population by the end of 10 years. This, in the opinion of these scholars, was further compounded by the Committee's recommendations against indigenous systems of medicine and for the abolition of the system of licentiate medical practitioners (Gautam and Shyamprasad, 2010).

The actual position is, however, that the Committee stood for universal coverage from the very outset, limited though their proposals were due to the constraints of resources. Speaking about its short-term plan, the Committee said:

> We wish to make it clear that the proposals that will be discussed in the succeeding paragraphs embody recommendations which are intended to supplement and not supplant the existing health facilities in the areas where our scheme will be introduced. We consider moreover, that our recommendations constitute an irreducible minimum, and, were it not for the limitation imposed by the inadequacy of staff and funds, we should unhesitatingly have proposed a more comprehensive scheme than the one indicated below (Government of India., 1946, Vol. II, p. 37).

The truth is that the Committee to its credit never lost sight of the need for universalization of health care. It put this on record in wholly unambiguous terms:

> We have come to the conclusion that the new health services, in howsoever attenuated a form they may be started, should be initiated on as wide a territorial basis as possible. We feel that, for the purpose of demonstrating the resulting improvement in the public health of a province as a whole, the application of our proposals in every district, though it may be over a limited area in each to begin with, will be more effective than concentration of effort in one or two small areas in the province (Ibid., Vol. II, p. 38).

Where Did the Committee Fail?

As is the wont with all great things, they need to be measured against equally high yardsticks. The Committee is as monumental in its failures as in its achievements. Just as the positive recommendations of the Committee were rooted in the objective social and political conditions of the time, its failings are also no abstractions and are firmly rooted in the political character of the governance paradigm that existed in India around the time of the

Committee's deliberations. The failures of the Committee could be many, perhaps even in excess of its achievements cited earlier; however, we shall dwell here on those that had the most far-reaching impact on the development of health services in India. A committee of such cardinal importance as the Bhore Committee cannot but be held responsible for the consequences of its recommendations.

It must be borne in mind that the Sirs, Colonels, Khan Bahadurs, and Dewan Bahadurs on the Committee were no radicals. They were persons in positions of power and well ensconced in the colonial apparatus. Apart from the political compulsion of having to deal with the rising aspirations of the people, their vision went only as far as the ruling apparatus of the day permitted and was marred by colonial attitudes towards the people at large.

The Choice of the Health care Model

Before arriving at its scheme for the development of health services in India, the committee thoroughly studied the 'modem trends in the organization of health services' across the world in order to choose a model for India (Government of India, 1946, Vol. II, pp. 6-16). Broadly, it narrowed down to two models to choose from: the 'Welfare State' model as it had come into existence in the UK and the model of 'Health as a Right' that existed in the Soviet Union. We need only elaborate at some length on what the committee itself said about the difference between the two. Regarding the attitude of the Soviet government towards the health of the people, quoting Prof. Henry Sigerist, it said:

> Health is one of the goods of life to which man has a right; wherever this concept prevails the logical sequence is to make all measures for the protection and restoration of health accessible to all, free of charge; medicine like education is then no longer a trade, it becomes a public function of the State (Ibid., Vol. II, p. 10).

Further elaborating on the implications of the 'Health as a Right' model the Committee observed:

> This conception of health as a public function has resulted in the development of a coordinated scheme of preventive and curative health services, which exists in no other country, and in the recognition

> of the need for providing an environment which will enable the body to remain healthy and to resist disease. For this reason the control of housing, of industrial conditions, and other aspects of life, comes under the care of the People's Commissariat of Public Health (Government of India, 1946, Vol. II, p. 10).

The pro-people character of the latter model of health care is elaborated as follows:

> The structure of the Soviet medical system follows the general administrative structure of the country. In order that planning may be complete for the whole state it is controlled on the one hand by the People's Commissariat of Health, on the other hand by health committees and health nuclei organized in every factory, on every one of the large collective farms, and in every district. The one form of control is the natural outcome of the recognition that health protection is a function of the state; the other is the logical outcome of the principle that the workers themselves must take an active part in the protection of their own health. The system as it now stands is therefore not one forced on either the people of Russia or the medical profession by a particular group or class, but has had the active support and criticism of those interested in the service either as the purveyors of medical treatment or as the consumers of medical care (Ibid., Vol. II, p. 11).

The 'Welfare State' model, on the other hand, is heavily dependent on the initiative of the state in ensuring the physical and economic access to universal health care. People are reduced to being mere recipients of health care with little active day-to-day control over it.

Given these options, the Committee consciously chose the 'Welfare State' model. Proposing anything less than that which was being implemented in the UK virtually at the same time would have been rejected outright by the people. The people thus were segregated from the process of implementation of their own welfare and the nature of the Indian state, constrained as it was by the colonial institutions of governance and a colonial mindset even after 1947, led to the state straying away from its declared objectives.

The failure to adopt the 'Health as a Right' approach was the first major flaw of the Bhore Committee.

Lack of Ideological Conviction in Proposing Universally Free Health care

We feel that a very large section of the people are living below the normal subsistence level and cannot afford as yet even the small contribution that an *insurance scheme* will require. We therefore consider that medical benefits will have, in any case, to be supplied free to this section of the population *until* at least its economic condition is materially improved.... We consider, therefore, that *for the present* medical services should be free to all without distinction and that the contributions from those who can afford to pay should be through the channel of general and local taxation (Government of India, 1946, Vol. II, p. 14; authors' emphasis).

It is very evident from the statement made earlier that the Committee's position against an imposition of 'user fees' in health services was more due to the expediency of the poverty of the people at that time rather than any ideological commitment towards provision of free health care. In this sense, the Committee left a toehold for later attempts to provide a foothold to user charges in health policy.

Imposition of the Western Model of Health care

It is hardly a secret that the Indian systems of medicine were allowed to languish during the colonial period, which had resulted in their becoming scientifically stagnant. Nonetheless, the practitioners of Indian systems of medicine, whatever their drawbacks, continued to command a huge clientele in vast parts of India both among illiterates and the intelligentsia. This, however, did not impress upon the Committee that they should consider any role for the indigenous systems in the future organization of health services in India; rooted as their convictions were in the positivist notions of biomedicine. They said:

> It was not until the middle of the 19th century that medical science became firmly established on a secure foundation. The invention of the compound microscope, the rapid development of Organic Chemistry and latterly of Bio-Chemistry and Bio-Physics have led to such an advance that we can say with truth that 95% of the total corpus of knowledge 'With regard to the working of the human body has been obtained within the lifetime of men who are still with us (Ibid., Vol. II, p. 456).

It was their firm belief that:

> Public health or preventive medicine, which must play an essential part in the future of medical organization, is not within the purview of the indigenous systems of medical treatment as they obtain at present (Ibid., Vol. II, p. 455).

Further:

> No system of medical treatment, which is static in conception and practice and does not keep pace with the discoveries and researches of scientific workers the world over, can hope to give the best available ministration to those who seek it (Government of India, 1946, Vol. II, p. 455).

The degeneration of the indigenous systems of medicine brought about by particular social, economic, and political conditions led the committee to virtually declare them to be 'unscientific', rather than propose ways and means of isolating and developing the scientific content of these systems in order that they might better serve the millions who continued to have faith in them. Such a contemptuous view was in no way different from the attitude of our colonial masters towards these systems and was compounded by the fact that not even one representative of these systems was on the Committee.

Further insult to injury was added by the recommendation that there should only be one category of highly trained doctor and that the licentiate system of medical practice should be abolished. They said:

> Having regard to the limited resources available for the training of doctors, it would be to the greater ultimate benefit of the country if those resources were concentrated on the production of only one and that the most highly trained type of doctor, which we have termed the 'basic' doctor (Ibid., Vol. II, p. 340).

The Report has considerable intellectual depth and grasp of the socio-economic realities, and suggests that the class background of the medical graduates passing out from the then existing medical colleges and the fact that these urban, and at that time purely upper class graduates, would be extremely resistant to manning the health services in the extremely impoverished countryside would not have been lost on the members. It is relevant to remember here that all policies for affirmative action notwithstanding, the élitist class character of the medical profession in India remains unchanged to the present time. The Bhore Committee contributed to fortifying these élitist credentials by recommending that:

> There should hereafter be a single portal of entry into the medical professions and that portal should be the universities. . . . We are confirmed in this view by the reasons advanced by the Inter Departmental Committee (the Good Enough Committee) on Medical Education in Great Britain in support: of University Medical Education (Government of India, 1946, Vol. II, p. 342).

The honourable members of the committee could not have been so naive as to not have realized that at that point in time it was largely the élite who could afford a university education for their children. The Committee could perhaps have cherished the misplaced hope that the social orientation of medical education would somehow right this, which obviously did not happen. Such ahistorical, colonial, and élitist policy orientation is at the root of the development of the entrepreneurial model of Western-oriented technological health care that privileges curative over preventive care and cities over towns, besides making the provision of health-care expensive and perennially dependent on the West. This model was more suited to Western rather than the indigenous health-care needs. It is little wonder then that Indian medical graduates have migrated in their droves to keep the health care systems of the US and UK afloat (Gautam and Shyamprasad, 2010). It is the oppressed poor who have had to pay the price of such a policy

It is not as if alternatives did not exist or were not proposed: on the contrary, the sub-committee on National Health of the National Planning Committee of the Indian National Congress, which was chaired by Col. S.S. Sokhey, proposed a more self-reliant path of health development suited to the specific conditions of development in India. The Sokhey Committee emphasized:

> From the standpoint of reorganizing the medical education of the health personnel in the country, Indian universities have almost all been devoted to medical science and research as taught in the West in all its branches . . . . If medical advice and treatment to the mass of the people is to be provided on the necessary scale free of charge, the National Plan will have to bring the indigenous Vaidya, Hakim, or

> Dai into line with more elaborately or pretentiously trained physician or surgeon. gynecologist or obstetrician. It is more a matter of the technique particularly in the case of the last named and certain precautions by way of cleanliness, than a matter of the actual drugs or appliances used (Sokhey Committee, 1948: 35).

While not discounting the importance of the modern technique and latest appliances, the Sokhey Committee said:

> These, however, must be made or found in the country in an ever-increasing degree. An important sector of the Plan will no doubt, have to be the provision, from the country's own resources, of all the drugs, medicines, appliances and instruments in safeguarding the health of the nation (Sokhey Committee. 1948: 35).

It is important to note that the policy framework of the Bhore Committee was approved by 11 of the 16 Indians on it, and among them were such 'nationalist' leaders as Dr B.C. Roy. This in itself bears testimony to the fact that the governance paradigm post-1947 was in essence the continuation of the colonial paradigm with the 'brown sahib' replacing the 'white sahib'; a truth that we shall see being borne out more fully in the recommendations on population policy.

Giving a Fillip to Vertical Health Programmes

Although the Bhore Committee adopted an epidemiological and systemic approach to public health, many of its recommendations for disease control ended up laying the ground for implementation of a series of what are now called vertical disease control programmes, beginning immediately after independence. With the benefit of hindsight we now know that these vertical programmes proved to be a major hindrance in the composite development of the general health services in India. Of the different health programmes we mention here, are the recommendations made for the control of malaria and tuberculosis.

The Committee fully endorsed the views of the Director, Malaria Institute of India, seeking a vertical approach to malaria control; he said, 'an essential preliminary to the successful control of malaria in India is the formation of an adequately staffed permanent malaria organization in each province, the activities of which should be linked with those of the central organization of the Government of India'. (Government of India, 1946, Vol. IV, p. 34)

The Committee said,

> Our recommendations, therefore include the establishment of anti-malaria organizations in the provinces as well as the strengthening of the staff of the Malaria Institute of India in order to enable it to fulfil its important tasks of advising provincial administrations in the development of anti-malaria measures, of coordinating such work in the provinces and of training the higher types of malaria personnel for the country as a whole.
>
> This was accompanied by recommendations for vertical management of the supply of drugs, appliances, and other equipment. The emphasis given to the use of insecticides over public health measures such as drainage of swamps, public health engineering, and general sanitary measures gives away the technocentric bias of the Committee (Government of India, 1946, Vol. IV, pp. 35-6).

Similarly, for comprehensive and integrated service for tuberculosis, the formation of a 'tuberculosis organization' comprising the following components was proposed:

> '(1) A domiciliary service, (2) clinics, (3) hospitals, (4) after-care colonies, (5) homes for the incurable and, in addition (6) certain ancillary services.' Five Year Plan-wise expansion in the clinical services for tuberculosis was also proposed (Ibid., Vol. IV, pp. 36-7).

India did launch soon after the transfer of power a massive military-like campaign in the name of the 'National Malaria Control Programme 'which was followed by the equally grandiose 'National Malaria Eradication Programme'. Though unsuccessful in achieving its objectives, the programmes did reduce the malaria public health problem considerably, but left the general health services emasculated and India having to continue to live with malaria in the absence of the more fundamental public health measures.

The other vertical programme that played truant with the health services was the massive family planning programme.

Views on Population Policy

One of the most central questions in development policy is how we view the people: whether they are the motive force for change or are they a part of the problem. Deciding on this determines the orientation we adopt in instituting development policies, that is, the poor, impoverished, illiterate, and diseased people are the muck that needs to be cleared and hence the programmes for education, health care, housing, nutrition, etc., or the poor are seen as long-suffering victims of social, political, and economic injustice and therefore the most urgent need is to dedicate ourselves to ameliorating their suffering. While the former may result in some improvement, it is the latter that results in palpable improvement in the lives of people.

That in the case of the Bhore Committee the former is the case is given away by its views in the chapter entitled 'The Population Problem' (Ibid., Vol. II, pp. 477-89), that is, to say that people are part of the problem. The Committee has adopted a belligerently Malthusian position at a time when Malthus had long been discredited in his own country. We feel obliged here to let the Committee express itself in its own words. It said:

> The history of the growth of population in India, therefore, seems to illustrate the contention of Malthus that disease and famine impose checks on an unlimited growth of population (Government of India, 1946, Vol. II, pp. 477-78).

What emerges is that disease and famine are not to be regarded as causes of human suffering but as instruments that maintain a 'check' on the population. We can understand that the Committee did not have the gumption to indict the colonial loot of India in any way, but here it has been seen fit to, in a way, mock the suffering of the people. Most shockingly the Committee stated:

> A reduction in the rate of growth of population may be brought about by permitting the death rate in the community to rise. Our social instincts militate against this.... One of the objectives universally accepted in all civilized countries is reduction of morbidity and mortality in the community. We have, therefore, to tum to other means for decreasing the rate of growth of the population (Ibid., Vol. II, pp. 483-4).

It almost appears that but for the ' social instincts' brought to bear by 'civilized countries', the Committee might well have recommended population reduction by 'permitting the death rate in the community to rise'. How else do we understand such a thought process on the part of a Committee charged with the task of improving the people's health?

Intentional Limitation of Families

Here the Committee's sheer contempt for the people and basal thinking with respect to the 'population question' seems to have known no limits. It writes:

> If we believe that limitation of families is advisable, we should first ask ourselves the question whether it is possible that this could be secured through self-control. Our answer must be, we fear, not to any material extent. A limited number of individuals may be undersexed or may, by nature, be so constituted that they can sublimate most of their sexual urge into intellectual, artistic or other creative channels. But the large majority of mankind, while they may be able to convert a part of their sexual impulse into activities useful to the community, will still have to find satisfaction in the sexual act itself.

In the Committee's opinion, birth control through 'positive means' was the only option (Government of India, 1946, Vol. II, pp. 483-4). Thankfully it did not suggest what these 'positive means' could be.

It is more than a curious coincidence that former health minister, Gulam Nabi Azad, had this to suggest for controlling the population of the country:

> If there is electricity in every village, then people will watch TV till late at night and then fall asleep. They won't get a chance to produce children.... When there is no electricity there is nothing else to do but produce babies (Blakely, 2009).

There is a more fundamental bond between the two statements: the bond of the colonial arrogance of the 'brown sahibs'. All science, all caution, all niceties and restraint were thrown to the wind in commenting thus on the character of the impoverished:

> A birth control campaign has certain inherent dangers.... Contraceptive practices are, therefore, more likely to be used by the more successful and intelligent sections of the community than by those who are improvident and mentally weak. It may also be mentioned that a certain number of defects and diseases are known to be heritable. These include . . . . the classes which possess many of

> these undesirable characteristics are known to be generally improvident and prolific. A continued high birth-rate among these classes, if accompanied by a marked fall in the rate of growth of the more energetic, intelligent and ambitious sections of the population, which make much the largest contribution to the prosperity of the country, may be fraught with serious consequences to national welfare (Government of India, 1946, Vol. II, p. 487).

The members of the Bhore Committee recommended legalization of 'voluntary sterilization' and advocated a fully-fledged 'eugenic programme' to improve the 'future composition of the community' as had been so successfully done by man in the case of different species of plants and animals (Ibid., Vol. II, pp. 488-9).

If the post-1947 experience is anything to go by, then it appears that the views of the Bhore Committee on the population question seem to have had an overbearing influence vis-à-vis its other recommendations. India was the first country in the world to launch a family planning programme.

Conclusion

The struggle for the improvement of the health services in India is an ongoing struggle of the people. The recommendations of the Bhore Committee have an enduring value in this context. Both the positive as well as the negative features of the Committee have a basis in the objective historical and political conditions of the time of its deliberations. Unfortunately, the failure of the health policy paradigm in India post-1947, especially the developments after the introduction of the World Bank-guided health reforms resulting in non-fulfilment of promises made at the time of independence, makes the positive recommendations of the Committee seem even more remarkable.

The analysis here has important implications for policy-making in the field of health. The fact that India has not even succeeded in achieving the targets set out in the short-term plan of the Committee, which were to have been achieved by the beginning of the 1980s, demands renewed vigour in the planned expansion of integrated, that is, preventive, promotive, curative, and rehabilitative health services, especially in the rural areas. It is a matter of great concern that some of the most fundamental principles of public health planning, that is, the epidemiological approach, a systems approach to health care and provision for training of public health personnel, which were espoused in the recommendations of the Committee, are missing in the planning of India's most ambitious health plan of recent times, that is, the NRHM which has since been converted to National Health Mission (NHM).

Apart from this, the pitfalls of the techno-centric approach in health planning geared towards expansion of costly curative health care, on one hand, and, on the other, technology-driven vertical disease control programmes, are clearly shown by our analysis. These remain potent threats to the wholesome development of health-care services in India to this day. There is a need to sublimate technology to the requirements of the people rather than sublimating people to the requirement of preconceived technological solutions offered by policy-planners.

The greatest threat, however, is the continuance of the colonial governance paradigm in India post-1947. That it comes packaged in the form of apparently liberal bourgeoisie democracy makes it more insidious, surreptitious but no less dangerous. This fact highlights that the struggle for development of pro-people health services in India is in the main a political struggle. Academics, health planners, and health activists need to be aware of the class alignment of forces in this struggle. While pushing for pragmatic health reforms in view of the present alignment of class forces, they should seek to emphasize the need for a political struggle to remedy this alignment.

REFERENCES

Abel-Smith, Brian (1992): 'The Beveridge Report: Its Origins and Outcomes', *International Social Security Review*, Vol. 45(1-2): 5-16.

Banerji, D. (2005): Politics of Rural Health in India, *International Journal of Health Services*, Vol. 35(4): 783-96.

Blakely, R. (2009): 'Ghulam Nabi Azad Says Late-Night TV Will Help Slow India's Birth Rate', *Sunday Times*, July 13.

Chopra, P.N., B.N. Puri, M.N. Das, A.C. Pradhan (2005): 'Civil Disobedience Movement' in 1930-34, in *A Comprehensive History of India, Modern India*, Sterling Publishers Private Limited, New Delhi, p. 247.

Dae, D.K., and A. Vanna, (1998): 'The Armed Police in the British Colonial Tradition: The Indian Perspective', *Policing: An International Journal of Police Strategies & Management,* Vol. 21(2), 354-67.

Globalsecurity.org. (2010): 'Regiments' in *Military.* Available from: htlp://www. globalsecurity.org/military/word/india/rgt.htm, accessed on October 22, 2010.

Government of India (1946): *Health Survey and Development Committee,* Vols. I, II and IV, Recommendations (New Delhi: Government of India).

Government of India (2005): *National Rural Health Mission (2005-2012) Mission Document* (New Delhi: Ministry of Health and Social Welfare).

Gautam, M., and K.M. Shyamprasad (2010): 'The "Basic" Doctor for Rural India: A Failed Promise?', *Economic & Political Weekly,* Vol. 45(38): 25-9.

Indian Courts. (2009): About Indian Penal Code. Available from: http://www.ipc.inI, accessed on October 21, 2010.

Pylee, M.V. (2002): *An Introduction to the Constitution of India* (5th edn.) (Delhi: Vikas Publishing House).

Singh, A. Imler (1985): 'Keeping India in the Commonwealth: British Political and Military Aims, 1947-49', *Journal of Contemporary History,* Vol. 20(3): 469-81.

Sokhey Committee (1948): *Sub-Committee on National Health, National Planning Committee* (Bombay: Vora and Co.).

The Hindu (2010): NAC Recommendations on Food Security Bill, October 25.

2

Of the Relationship Between Population and Development: Stop Vilifying the People*

Introduction

In the first chapter we dealt with the Bhore Committee Report that laid down the format of development of public health services in the country. Among other recommendations of the Committee we also had 'only a glimpse' of what the Committee thought on the population question, and among that regarding the poorest of the poor. Indeed, as the subsequent developments show, population has become the easiest alibi for placing the responsibility for all measure of social problems at the doorstep of the people. It would be prudent in that case to first clarify the relationship between population and development before we go any further in examining the way the health system has shaped in the country.

The world population touched seven billion some time ago and, as expected, there was an outpouring of concern over how the burgeoning population was the greatest stumbling block for our development. The relationship between population and development has been viewed as a one-way ticket where population is an independent variable and 'development' a

---

* This chapter had earlier been published as an article in the *Journal of Health Management*. The full reference of which is - Bajpai, Vikas, Suman Bhasker, Anoop Saraya (2012): 'Of the Relationship Between Population and Development: Need to Stop Vilifying the People', *Journal of Health Management*, 14(3): 329-340.

dependent one. This perception of population is well-entrenched not only among the laity but even amongst policy-makers. The result is that the people, who suffer due to lack of development, are often held responsible for their own impoverishment. The simplistic logic is that the population of the poor keeps increasing and that the government obviously cannot provide for so many people. Hence, the emphasis on family planning measures to restrict the population growth.

Experience from across the world indicates that populations in different countries have stabilized quite independently of population control measures. Subtle or overt coercion or incentives and disincentives have always formed a part of the family planning programme in India. The emphasis devoted to a family planning programme often led to a distortion of health priorities, and yet the programme has had very little to show in terms of substantial gains. Equally, India's development has not resulted in any substantive improvement in the quality of lives of the majority of our people. This is easily attested to by India's human development indices, which are among the worst in the world, with large areas faring worse than even many sub-Saharan countries.

Under such conditions, the continuance of the traditional approach to the question of 'population control' spells further disaster. There is clearly a need to review the one-way conceptualization of the relationship between population and development, and consequently reorient the population policy. As we shall see in this chapter, population growth has played a very important role in the development of human civilization and there is no reason for us to vilify the poor for the growth in their numbers.

The Ideological Roots of This Vilification

Much of the population bashing discourse on the population question is inspired directly or indirectly by the theory of population that was propounded by Thomas Malthus in 1798. Malthus propounded that the population increases in geometrical proportion, while the means of subsistence, chiefly food, increase in arithmetical proportion, and that the power of the population is immensely more than the capacity of the earth to provide for its subsistence. Under these circumstances the population is kept in check by what he called *'positive means'* such as famines, disease, and pestilence (Malthus 1998).

His assertions about the growth-rates of population and food were not supported by any empirical evidence. It is perhaps *because* of the lack of a refined scientific logic and the simplistic intuitiveness of his proposition that Malthus continues to inspire many people to this day. Importantly, Malthus did not confine himself to prophesy about population growth alone, but even foreclosed the possibility of a society in which things could be any better than his apocalyptic pronouncement stated. He said:

> This natural inequality of the two powers of population and of production in the earth ... I see no way by which man can escape from the weight of this law which pervades all animated nature. No fancied equality, no agrarian regulations in their utmost extent, could remove the pressure of it even for a single century. And it appears, therefore, to be decisive against the possible existence of a society, all the members of which should live in ease, happiness, and comparative leisure; and feel no anxiety about providing the means of subsistence for themselves and families (Malthus 1998: 5).

History bears testimony to the fact that the populations across the world have grown enormously since Malthus made his pronouncements without any of his prophecies being borne out. Even as Malthus stood thoroughly discredited in the Western world, the perceived threat of a population explosion in the developing world led to a resurrection of his ideas after the Second World War in the form of neo-Malthusianism.

It is important to point out here that concerns regarding population growth have always been an elitist agenda where it is invariably the population of the poor that is a matter of concern. Such a discourse is like the dialogue of the deaf talking down to the dumb, where the elite do all the talking without having to listen to the poor whose population growth they are talking about; the poor barely have a say.

Malthus's concern was entirely about the population of the poor working classes of the UK: similarly, such concerns in the US were also about the populations of the poor. Decrying the race suicide of upper-class women, President Theodore Roosevelt said in 1907:

> ... the greatest problem of civilization is to be found in the fact that the well-to-do families tend to die out . . . the prudent and thoughtful (whose children the race needs) would be the ones to practise birth control while knowledge of contraception was unlikely to affect the fertility of the reckless lower classes (Hodgson and Watkins, 1997: 5).

Economic growth and progress in the human development indices of the West, in which the transfer of wealth from the Third World had a big role, led to conditions in which the population of the underprivileged sections of the people was no longer perceived to be a problem in these countries. The attention thus shifted to the population of the poor in the Third World.

Private foundations, like the Rockefeller and Ford Foundations, were to become the fountainheads of elite interests on the population question. These foundations contributed hugely to the establishment of 'population centres' in major US universities and, through them, 'an international academic and policy elite invested in fertility reduction as a national development strategy' (Hodgson and Watkins 1997: 6; Hartmann 2006). In the words of Caldwells, an 'ideological conversion' of foreign students who were trained in demography at these centres was carried out where they were persuaded of the urgent need to reduce birth rates' in their countries (Hartmann 2006). It is not very difficult to gauge that these population experts trained in the US shared much the same perception as that of their white teachers towards the poor in their own countries.

The international agencies also imbibed this elitist discourse on population growth. The 1987 report of the United Nations World Commission on Environment and Development (WCED) entitled, *Our Common Future,* spoke of the devastating effects of population, 'Those who are poor and hungry will often destroy their immediate environment in order to survive. They will cut down forests: then livestock will overgraze grasslands; they will overuse marginal lands and in growing numbers they will crowd into congested cities' (WECD, 1987: 6). The report identifies 'environmental stress' and 'environmental refugees' as an important source of conflict.

In the post-Cold War era, the rhetoric around the population issue was reified into a new 'security threat', and hence a reason for the continued deployment of the US forces beyond its borders.

In the *National Security Strategy of Engagement and Enlargement*, of 1994-5, the US administration stated that 'large-scale environmental degradation, exacerbated by rapid population growth, threatens to undermine political stability in many countries and regions' (White House 1995: 7).

Till as recently as 2003, a report entitled, *The Security Demographic: Population and Civil Conflict After the Cold War*, published by Population Action International, a Washington-based think tank, identified the youth bulge (a high proportion of young males in a given population), rapid urban growth, competition for crop land and fresh water, and AIDS-related deaths in the prime of life as factors contributing to increased risk of civil conflict (Cincotta et al. 2003: 7).

Superimposed over these fears are concerns about environmental degradation that may be caused by advances in technology, including the technology that resulted in lowering the death rates which thus resulted in an increase in population. However, these demonizing constructs of population growth prove to be fortresses built of sand once we care to look at the historical trends of high population growth and seek to understand the factors that have affected these trends.

Historical Trends in Population Growth

Tables 1 and 2 present the broad trends in the growth of world population. Table 1 provides data on the quantum of population growth associated with different phases of development of human civilization identified by their principal mode of production, while Table 2 provides a comparison of the relative growth-rates of population between European settlements (Europe, the Americas, Australia, etc.), Asia and Africa in different time periods.

Table 1 clearly shows that the overall growth of the world population and the rates of growth in population increased as the means of production in the society advanced. Improved means of production resulted in new relations of production, much greater production, and more efficient distribution of produce, thereby enabling the transition of human civilization to a higher stage of development. The different phases of development in the means of production also determined the ability of the society to fight

Table 1: The Historical Phases of Population Growth

Time Period	*Human Population (millions)*	*Average Growth Rate/1,000 {% in brackets)*	*Doubling Time*
1. Pre-agricultural era: hunters and gatherers (35,000-10,000 BC)	6	0.08 per 1,000 (0.008%)	8,000 to 9,000 years
2. Spread of agricultural societies (10,000 BC-0)	252	0.37 per 1,000 (-0.037%)	1,854 years
3. Further development of predominantly rural societies (0-1750 AD)	771	0.64 per 1,000 (–0.064%)	1,083 years
4. The industrial revolution (1750-1950)	2,520	6 per 1.000 (0.6%)	116 years
5. Further Industrial/ Technoligical advanced 1950-2000	6,235	18.1 per 1,000 (1.81%)	38 years

Source: Livi-Bacci {1997), quoted in Wuyts (1998)

Table 2: Differential Growth Rates in Population

Period	*World*	*European Settlements*	*Asia*	*Africa*
1000-1750	0.13	0.13	0.14	0.09
1750-1800	0.44	0.64	0.49	-0.21
1800-1850	0.50	0.81	0.42	0.21
1850-1900	**0.64**	**1.10**	**0.44**	**0.37**
1900-1930	0.76	1.09	0.50	0.96
1930-1960	1.34	1.02	1.52	1.63
1960-1990	1.89	0.63	2.43	2.47
1990-2025 (pr.)	1.30	0.76	1.17	2.84

Source: Hayami (1997), quoted in Wuyts (1998)

disease, natural disasters, and other causes of death, as developments in science and technology accompanied the development of the means of production. Thus, every distinct phase in human civilization was characterized by its distinctive balance between death and birth rates and a growth rate of population determined by the means to sustain the population. Fig. 1 graphically represents the increase in human population during the different phases of human civilization.

As against the claims by Malthus, Marx very aptly stated that 'every special historic mode of production has its own special laws of population, historically valid, within its limit alone' (Kuznetsov 1957: 8). This serves to highlight that the size of population is clearly a dependent variable which is determined by the level of development of the society and the manner in which its resources are distributed among people.

Fig. 1: Growth of Human Population Through History

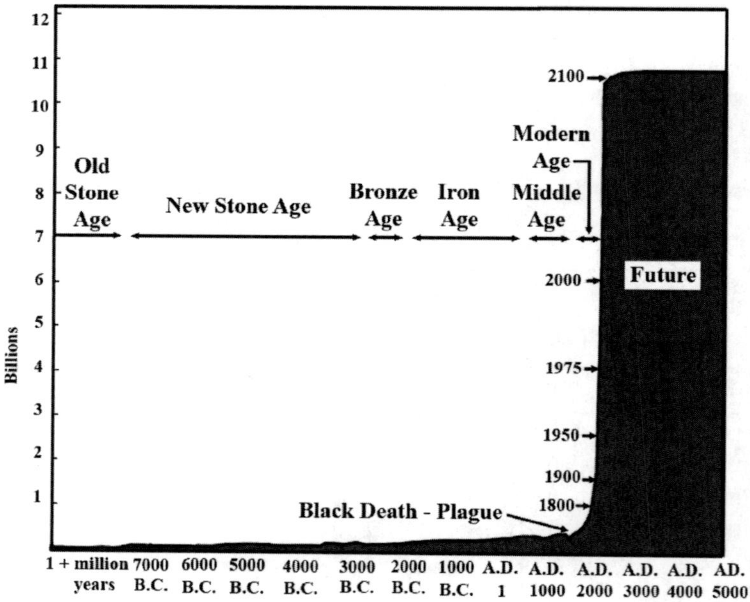

Source: Population Reference Bureau; and United Nations, World Population Projections to 2100 (1998)

Table 2 clearly shows that high rates of population growth are not peculiar to the developing countries of Asia and Africa alone, and that the countries of the developed world have witnessed periods of high population growth till not very long ago. In fact, it is only in the 20th century that the population growth-rates began to decline in these countries and it was not till the 1960s that these growth-rates saw real deceleration. This happened as a consequence of a high level of well-being of the people at large with the establishment of welfare states in the industrialized world that led to huge declines in poverty, illiteracy, and ill-health of the people.

Importantly, the real jump in the growth-rates of population in the countries of Asia and Africa occurred only after the Second World War, when public health and other welfare measures were introduced for the first time after many of these countries gained political independence. The long period of colonialism had left the economies of these countries battered and even after independence; the condition of dependence on the West of most of these countries has only enabled a very slow pace of decline in poverty, illiteracy, and ill-health of their people. Nevertheless, the important message that emerges is that development in the conditions of the lives of the people has always preceded population stabilization.

Unscrambling the Population Myth

It is feared that population growth will lead to a rapid depletion of resources for human sustenance, causing environmental degradation and increased human suffering. The world has already witnessed its population increase many times since the industrial revolution in the UK; it will be interesting to see whether the empirical data support these fears of population growth.

The relationship between the environmental impact of population, human affluence, and technologies has been conceptually expressed by the equation, I = PAT, where I is the measure of environmental impact; P is the population; A stands for human affluence, a surrogate for per capita production or per capita consumption; and T, denoting technology, is a measure of the impact of technology per unit of production or consumption (Chertow et al. 2008). The IPAT equation implies that if everything else remains the same, then the population, human affluence, and technology will act as multipliers for the environmental impact. The higher the population, the greater willl be the consumption, and the greater affluence with economic development will lead to higher human production and consumption. Technology can impact in different ways; it can be highly resource intensive, but by improving efficiency, the per capita impact on the environment can be reduced. The higher the overall environmental impact of population, affluence, and technology, the less will be the level of human well-being. The IPAT equation has been used to demonstrate that the present levels of human production and consumption are not sustainable in the long ran unless the human population decreases and cleaner and greener technologies are developed (Goklany 2009).

The empirical evidence does not however seem to bear out these apprehensions. Using long-term cross-country data, it has been demonstrated that despite growth in population across the world, deployment of newer technologies and a rapid increase in consumption patterns associated with increased economic growth, human well-being has only increased to unprecedented levels, as can be witnessed from the trends across a variety of indicators, such declines in total fertility rates, increase in health adjusted life expectancy, infant mortality, and food availability (Goklany 2009).

Trends in Total Fertility Rates and Population Growth Rates

The original neo-Malthusian premise was that the population would grow exponentially. Even though it is now hypothesized that the world population is likely to stabilize at around nine billion by 2100 (O'Neill et al. 2004), the cultivated notion, as reflected through some of the reports mentioned earlier, the popular perception is that the continuing growth of human population willl inevitably result in a catastrophic finale. Fig. 2 shows the declining trends in the total fertility rates and population growth-rates with an increase in per capita gross domestic product (GDP) (an indicator of increased economic affluence) over a period of time (which can be a crude indicator of the secular advance of new technology). There is an unambiguous decline in total fertility rates and population growth-rates with increase in per capita GDP and advancements in technology, which contradicts the neo-Malthusian premise.

The relationship between economic affluence and total fertility rates and population growth-rates is mediated by a number of factors, only some of which are being identified here. Increasing economic prosperity means that the society is able to take better care of its people, especially the vulnerable groups such as the old and children. This serves to reduce the drive to have more children: one, because the parents are more certain that their children will

Fig. 2: Changes in Total Fertility Rates and Population Growth-Rates with Increasing GDP and Secular Advancement of Technology

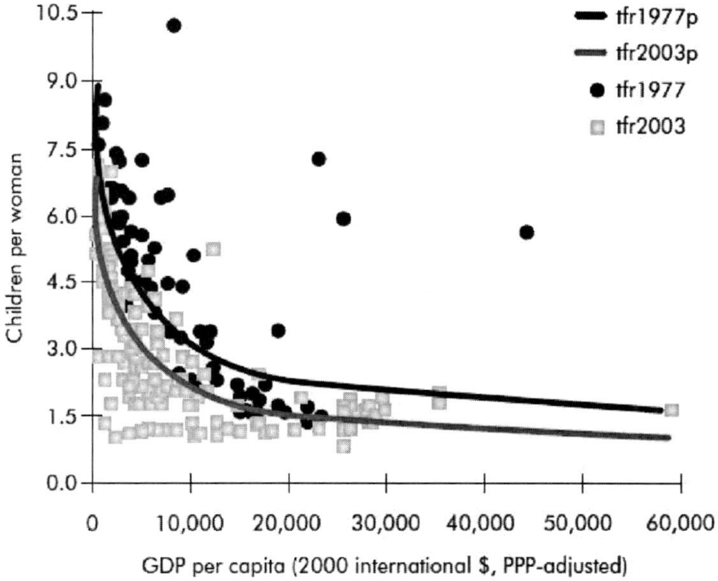

Source: Goklany (2007).
Note: tfr = total fertility rate, P = population growth rates

survive into adulthood; and second, because the children need not always be viewed as the only social insurance in old age when the society is able to provide better social security (Goklany 2009).

Richer societies are able to provide better educational and employment opportunities for women which tends to raise the age at marriage, and the increased opportunity costs to families with employed women due to frequent child-bearing serves as a disincentive for having more children. Education of women also has the effect of providing sanitary conditions for bringing up children and a better awareness of preventive health interventions such as breast-feeding and immunization.

Economic advancement and access to technology that comes with it, reduces the value of labour performed by children. This also reduces the impetus to have more children. Moreover, the economic and technological advancement of society means that the education and upbringing of children, in order to train them in the advanced methods of the society, becomes more expensive; this also serves as a disincentive for having more children (Goklany 2009). Most importantly, the greater well-being of society means that the aspirations of the people change as they have greater opportunities for their development, enabling them to move beyond the daily strife for bread and butter. This brings about a change in the traditional family structures and values such that fewer children are considered a desirable end.

The above-mentioned developments clearly show that one of the most fundamental fears of Malthus that greater prosperity of a society will only lead to people irresponsibly reproducing their numbers and thereby bringing about their own downfall has been thoroughly discredited. This clearly shows that the P in the IPAT equation is not exclusive of A and T. Much less than being an independent variable, it is clearly influenced by the overall development of a society.

However, it would be prudent to strike a cautionary note here, that is, that economic growth and increasing affluence will not in themselves pay all the above-mentioned dividends: they have to be wedded with principles of equity, social justice, and empowerment, which can be ensured only if the fruits of growth are distributed to the entire society rather than nurturing the mega profits of small sections of it. For a population to stabilize, it is important that women become equal members of the society and exercise full control over their bodies. In the absence of empowerment, education, and job opportunities for women may only add income generation as an extra burden over and above the burden of domestic work and strengthen their chains of bondage.

Trends in Human Well-Being

We need not need to prove here that over the years, affluence of even the poorest of countries has increased in terms of per capita GDP, and technological advances have increased the gobbling up of the earth's resources manifold; even so, this has not resulted in diminishing well-being of the people. Table 3 sets out the improvements in various parameters of human well-being over the years. There have been overall improvements in human well-being even for the developing and least developed countries which have witnessed high increases in the populations due to rapid declines in mortality rates and the high fertility of then predominantly younger populations.

However, it is important to note that these are only overall trends which in themselves conceal the marked inter-regional and intra-regional variations across caste, class, gender, ethnicity, etc. For example, in the 1980s, sub-Saharan Africa, and in the 1990s, the countries of the former Soviet Union witnessed deterioration in many of these development indicators due to floundering economies. Similarly, within a country like India, there remain large sections of the population that have slipped down the human development ladder, while a smaller section has seen improvements comparable to those of the First World, thereby pulling up the averages. Nevertheless, there has been a definite overall improvement.

Contrary to the neo-Malthusian view, many authors have identified population growth as being directly responsible for increasing the well-being and prosperity of societies (Boserup 1972; Madsen et al. 2010; Scott and Scherr 1999; Simon 1996). The basic contention of these authors is that the pressure on resources due to a growth of population leads to innovations in production techniques and technologies, leading to greater production of resources required for human welfare, and that such innovation is inexhaustible. Scott and Scherr (1999) have reported 70 empirical studies which document that population growth has not led to environmental degradation, decimation of forests, and uprooting of agriculture or of watersheds in the hills and mountains of developing countries.

By now, most of us who have been used to understanding population growth as the villain of the piece might begin wondering whether this chapter is arguing for the population control programme to be converted into a population decontrol programme and asking for a baby boom. That is certainly not the contention of this chapter. We know two things for certain: one, the earth's natural resources, if not very limited, are certainly not infinite; and second, that the tell-tale signs of environmental degradation are for real and that every country in the world is

Table 3: Improvement in Human Well-Being with Time (or Technological Change) and Economic Growth

Income (2000 international $)	*Daily Food Supplies Per Capita[a] (kcal)*		*Infant Mortality (per 1,000 live births)*		*Life Expectancy in Years*		*Tertiary Student Enrolment (%)*		*Access to Safe Water (%)*	
	1975	2002	1980	2003	1975	2003	1975	2002	1990	2002
$ 1 a day	1.652	1.818	355	207	40.7	44.6	0.9	1.5	39.1	41.7
$2 a **day**	**1.897**	**2,064**	**199**	**1 16**	**46.2**	**50.2**	**1.7**	**2.8**	**47.7**	**50.9**
$ 1.000 per year	2.009	2,175	154	90	48.7	52.7	2.3	3.8	52.2	55.7
$10,000 per year	2,825	2,991	23	13	67.2	7IJ	19.8	31.9	100.0	100.0
Average for low income countries[b]	2.027	2,390	147	52	49.2	58.0	2.4	6.6	53.0	66.3
World average[b]	2.540	2,863	44	17	60.8	68.5	9.4	22.8	80.3	97.4

Source: Goklany (2007).

Notes: (a) As given in the original source:

[a] Based on data from World Resources Institute's Earth Trends database, available at www.wri.org (accessed June 23, 2005), except as noted.

[b] Based on data from World Bank's World Development Indicators.

(b) The original author of this table based his calculations using data from World Bank, World Development Indicators, available at http://devdata.worldbank.org/dataonline (accessed July 12, 2005), except where noted.

liable to shortages of one kind or another: food especially is a resource that has become quite precarious in its availability over the past few years. The need to exercise caution becomes even more important when we find that some advocates of 'limitless bounties of mother earth and the ingenuity of the human race in adapting to population pressure' are unabashed proponents of free market capitalism, which we know, has caused enormous environmental damage in various parts of the world; more especially in the developing world.

In the context of how a reasonably long experience of the process of globalization and neoliberal economic reforms with unprecedented growth-rates of the economy coexisting with increasing socio-economic disparities, stagnant human development indicators, and increasing restlessness among large sections of the people, we can say with certainty that the current model of development has seriously undermined human well-being. Deprivation of a large section of the population directly undermines the 'human ingenuity' that has otherwise helped advance the well-being of the human race in the past.

A planned development policy based on principles of equity and social justice that prioritizes the needs and well-being of the people rather than profit maximization by a few is alone capable of judiciously exploiting the natural resources and ensuring their longevity. Planned development is the best surety for creating the material conditions in society that can help stabilize the population growth. In the light of the foregoing, it is imperative to understand what ought to be the components of our population policy.

For a Nuanced Understanding of Population Control

In the light of the above, the first and the most important fact to acknowledge is that rather than being an independent variable and having a negative impact on the socio-economic development of society, population is very much a dependent variable, the dynamics of which is heavily influenced by socio-economic development and the manner in which the social, economic, and political organization of the society mediates the relationship between people and resources. Second, rather than viewing population as 'a problem', it ought to be seen as a resource which, if properly developed, can immensely contribute to the enrichment of society in multifarious ways. In the context of the two stated requirements, the concept of unmet need needs to be expanded much beyond the narrow confines of fertility control measures to fulfil the unmet need for health care, food, housing, education, and employment.

Given this understanding, the first requirement of a comprehensive population policy is the creation of conditions which will enable all-round development of people to enable them to contribute to the development of the society to the best of their ability without the stigma of being called a 'problem'. Achieving this would require provision of satisfactory health care, education, housing, and employment opportunities to all. Second, integral to a population policy has to be adequate provision of family planning methods that will enable young men and women to regulate the growth of their families in a manner that is most conducive to their social and economic development.

Hence, the primary objective of the population policy shifts from that of 'stabilization of the population' to being 'the wholesome development of our human resource'. Our policy-planners are likely to jump at this to claim that this is precisely what they seek to achieve through the National Population Policy (NPP) 2000 (Government of India, 2000). Well, perhaps speaking generally about the population policy this may be true, but in terms of specifics, the NPP 2000 states:

> The *immediate objective* of the NPP 2000 is to address the unmet needs for contraception, health care infrastructure, and health personnel, and to provide integrated service delivery for basic reproductive and child health care. The *medium-term objective* is to bring the TFR to replacement levels by 2010, through vigorous implementation of inter-sectoral operational strategies. The *long-term objective* is to achieve a stable population by 2045, at a level consistent with the requirements of sustainable economic growth, social development, and environmental protection (Government of India, 2002).

Even though the 'National Socio-Demographic Goals for 2010' mentioned in the policy provide for improving health care and free and compulsory education up to the age of 14 years, most of the health interventions spoken of are related just to 'reproductive and child health'. The fourteenth and the last point in the goals speaks about bringing 'about convergence in implementation of related social sector programs so that family welfare becomes a people-centred programme'. Whatever may be the objectives of the policy, the overall thrust that emerges from a reading of the policy document is very much one of 'controlling the numbers'. That formulation and implementation of population policy is considered specifically the responsibility of the Ministry of Health, rather than that of all the ministries concerned with socio-economic development, is itself fraught with problems.

Concluding Remarks

If we have correctly understood that the path to population stabilization passes through the overall socio-economic development of the people, then it is obvious that the current population policy falls way short of achieving the targets set by it. This has indeed been the story of our population control programme since 1952.

An additional danger comes from the neoliberal development paradigm being currently pursued by the ruling elite. There is no need for us to draw inferences when the facts speak for themselves. In the last decade, India's economy has grown at an average of 8 per cent per annum and yet the percentage of GDP devoted to health, education and social welfare seems to have been frozen in time. Thanks to the deliberations of the National Advisory Council (NAC) earlier over the Food Security Bill, it has become an acknowledged fact that over 70 per cent of India's population is food insecure and yet it is acknowledged that the now enacted 'Food Security Act' adopt a minimalist position.

Such is the precarious position created by the current development policy paradigm that the government is itself having to acknowledge its devastating impact both on the people and the environment. The cancellation of approval for the setting up of an aluminium refinery by the Sterlite Group at Niyamgiri in Orissa and the adverse environmental impact report on the proposed POSCO steel plant in the same state by a committee of the central government are cases in point. According to one estimate, about 50 million people across India have been displaced due to various development projects since 1947. These features of the development policy in the country make the struggle of a proper population policy a part of the general democratic struggle of the people.

REFERENCES

Boserup, Ester (1972): *The Conditions of Agricultural Growth (*London: George Allen & Unwin).

Chertow, M., Cutler Cleveland and John Felleman (2008): 'IPAT equation', in Cutler J. Cleveland (ed.), *Encyclopedia of Earth (*Washington, DC: Environmental Information Coalition, National Council for Science and the Environment, retrieved from http://www.eoearth.oig/article/JJAT_equation. (First published in the *Encyclopedia of Earth,* on November 18, 2008.)

Cincotta, Richard P., Robert Engelman, and Daniele Anastasion (2003): *The Security Demographic: Population and Civil Conflict After the Cold War (*Washington. DC: Population Action International).

Goklany, I.M. (2007): *The Improving State of the World: Why We are Living Longer; Healthier, More Comfortable Lives on a Cleaner Planet (*Washington, DC: Cato Institute).

Goklany, I.M. (2009): 'Have Increases in Population, Affluence and Technology Worsened Human and Environmental Well-Being?' *The Electronic Journal of Sustainable Development,* Vol. 1(3).

Government of India (2000): *National Population Policy, 2000 (*New Delhi: Ministry of Health and Family Welfare).

Government of India (2002): *National Population Policy, 2002 (*New Delhi: Ministry of Health and Family Welfare).

Hartmann, B. (2006): 'Liberal Ends, Illiberal Means: National Security, "Eenvironmental Conflict" and the Making of the Cairo Consensus', *Indian Journal of Gender Studies,* 13(2), 196-227.

Hodgson, D., and Susan Cotts Watkins (1997): 'Feminists and Neo-Malthusians: Past and Present Alliances', *Population and Development Review,* 23(3), 469-523.

Kuznetsov, B. (1957): 'The Malthiusian Body', *International Affairs,* 3(2), 151-3.

Madsen, J.B., James B. Ang, and Rajabrata Banerjee (2010): 'Four Centuries of British Economic Growth: The Roles of Technology and Population', CAMA Working Papers 2010-18 (Australian National University: Centre for Applied Macroeconomic Analysis).

Malthus, T. (1998). *An Essay on the Principle of Population,* Electronic Scholarly Publishing Project, (London).

O'Neill, B.C., F.L. MacKellar, and W. Lutz (2004): 'Population, Greenhouse

Gas Emissions and Climate Change', in W. Lutz, W.C. Sanderson, and S. Scherbov (eds.), *The End of Population Growth in the 21st Century* (London: Earthscan), pp. 283-314. Population Reference Bureau; and United Nations, World Population Projections to 2100 (1998), quoted in 'Falkingham Jane'. The World at 7 Billion: Demographic Transition, Economic Development and the Demographic Dividend, School of Social Sciences, University of Southampton, Undated.

Templeton, S.R. and Sara J. Scherr (1999): 'Effects of Demographic and Related Microeconomic Change on Land Quality in Hills and Mountains of Developing Countries', *World Development*, 27(6), 903–18.

Simon, J. (1996): *The Ultimate Resource* (New Jersey: Princeton University Press).

White House (1995): 'National Security Strategy of Engagement and Enlargement, July 1994 and February 1995', in *Environmental Change and Security Project Report*, 1, (World Commission on Environment and Development (WCED), 1987), pp. 47-50 and *Our Common Future* (Oxford: Oxford University Press).

Wuyts, M. (1998): Malthus, Then and Now: The Novelty of Old Ideas on Population and Economy, Dies Natalis Address Delivered at the International Institute of Social Studies, Erasmus University of Rotterdam, The Hague, Netherlands, 8 October.

3

Landmarks in the Development of Health Care Services in India*

Introduction

Health care services in a country are influenced by its socio-economic development as well as political trends. The colonial domination by the British was largely responsible for the modernization of health care services in India. This influence remained even after independence in 1947.

Indian society is stratified into classes, castes and social groups based on ethnicity, race and gender. The aspirations of all these groups—often competing for a greater share—shape the developmental processes including health care institutions. Though policy-planners seek to reconcile these competing interests, the dominant sections corner the lion's share of invariably limited resources. This is reflected in the way health resources are used and appropriated.

Like competing social groups at the national level, unequal power relations exist among nations resulting in unequal distribution of international resources for health care. This too shapes health policies, and the development of health care systems in both the smaller and weaker nations.

---

* This chapter had initially been published as an article in the *National Medical Journal of India* and is being reproduced here with some modifications with the permission of the journal. The full reference of the earlier article is - Bajpai, Vikas, Anoop Saraya (2013): 'Development of Health care Services in India', *The National Medical Journal of India*, Vol. 26 (2): 240-245.

Thus, the development of health care services in a country needs to be understood as a process that takes shape under the influence of competing and contradictory aspirations of different sections of society and countries. We need to understand these influences to develop equitable health services in India.

Public Health Under The British

The Indian Medical Service of the East India Company acquired an all India character in April 1896, with the amalgamation of the Bengal Medical Service, the Madras Medical Service and the Bombay Medical Service (Mushtaq, 2009). The medical services under the British served their interests, i.e. ensuring the health of their troops and that of the European settlers, rather than the health needs of the local population. However, frequent outbreaks of disease in the general population due to poor sanitary conditions left British settlements vulnerable, forcing the British administration to take steps to control the epidemics as well as other public health measures. For example, the Royal Commission of 1859 recommended the establishment of a Commission of Public Health in each presidency and pointed to the need to improve sanitation to prevent epidemics in the general population, so that the health of the British Army could be better taken care of (Harrison, 1994). The Central Sanitary Department was formed in 1870, followed by sanitary departments in different provinces by 1879 (Mushtaq, 2009). The Vaccination Act (1880), the Births and Deaths Registration Act (1873) and the Epidemic Diseases Act (1897) were other such measures. In 1939, the Madras Public Health Act was passed, which was the first of its kind in India (Madras Public Health Act, 1939).

The Montgomery–Chelmsford Constitutional Reforms of 1919 led to the transfer of public health, sanitation and vital statistics to the provinces under the control of an elected minister. The Government of India Act, 1935 gave further autonomy to provincial governments. All health activities were categorized in three parts: federal, federal-cum-provincial and provincial (Park, 2007). This scheme continues till date.

With the British deciding after the Second World War to transfer power to the local leaders, plans were made for the development of health services in independent India. The most important development was the appointment of the Health Survey and Development Committee (popularly known as the Bhore Committee) in 1943 to survey the existing health structure in India and make recommendations for the future (Park, 2007). The recommendations made by this Committee are important in as much as they epitomized the hopes and aspirations of the people, and committed the government of independent India to the all round development of the health of the people.

The Bhore Committee

The landmark recommendations made by the Bhore Committee in 1946 continue to be relevant even today. The Committee said, 'Expenditure of money and effort on improving the nation's health is a gilt-edged investment which will yield not deferred dividends to be collected years later, but immediate and steady returns in substantially increased productive capacity. We need no further justification for attempting to evolve a comprehensive plan which must inevitably cover a very wide field and necessarily entail large expenditure, if it is to take into account all the more important factors which got the building up of a healthy, virile and dynamic people' (Government of India, 1946).

Committing the state as the chief guarantor of the health of its people, the Bhore Committee said: 'The idea that the state should assume full responsibility for all measures, curative and preventive, which are necessary for safeguarding the health of the nation, is developing as a logical sequence. The modern trend is towards the provision of as complete a health service as possible by the state and the inclusion, within its scope, of the largest possible proportion of the community' (Government of India, 1946).

The Bhore Committee epitomized an epidemiological approach to development of health services in conformity with the principles of social justice, equitable access, community participation, integration of preventive, promotive and curative services, and primacy to the needs of the rural people. There was a short-term plan and a long-term plan for developing the health infrastructure (Government of India, 1946). The Interim Government which was formed before independence, accepted the recommendations of the Bhore Committee.

Meanwhile, the sub-committee on health of the National Planning Committee of the Indian National Congress (Sokhey Committee) provided its own set of recommendations which underscored the direction given by the Bhore Committee. In addition, it stressed the need to integrate the indigenous systems of medicine within the mainstream to achieve self-sufficiency in health care (Sokhey Committee Report, 1948).

Health Services Since Independence

Post-independence, health planning became an integral part of planning for socio-economic development. Indian planners conceived the development of health services integrated with plans for tackling unemployment, malnutrition, social justice, housing and environmental sanitation (Banerji, 1985). However, this seemed difficult to achieve in practice.

In the two decades after 1947, health planning was done by way of schemes and programmes that were formulated as part of Five Year Plans. During this time several committees were formed to evaluate the achievements and failures of these programmes (Duggal, Undated). Some important landmarks are discussed.

Vertical Disease Control Programmes

Faced with a large burden of communicable diseases, limited resources and a need for rapid progress, there was impatience among health planners. Hence, a number of short-term measures were proposed for these problems, overlooking the need for overall socio-economic development of the people, as had happened in the West. This resulted in a series of techno-centric campaigns against malaria, smallpox, leprosy, filariasis, trachoma, cholera and for family planning. Large sums of money were made available for these programmes, at times at the cost of general medical services, in the hope of controlling or even eradicating these diseases (Banerji, 1985). The limitations of such an approach were apparent rather early. Even though the National Malaria Control Programme considerably brought down the incidence and prevalence of malaria, efforts to eradicate malaria through an eradication programme were ineffective due to inefficiency of general health services to be able to maintain the gains of the control programme. As a result, outbreaks of malaria continue to occur in different parts of the country till date. The leprosy eradication programme suffered a similar fate. India launched the National Leprosy Elimination Programme in 1993 to decrease the prevalence of leprosy to the WHO defined target of <1 per 10,000 population. This target was achieved in 2005. However, India still has 64% of prevalence and 78% of new case detection worldwide (Jain, 2012). About 7 years after achieving the WHO target of leprosy elimination, there are reports of leprosy increasing again (Mehta et al., 2009; Nelson, 2012).

The work done by tuberculosis workers was a notable exception to this general trend. The National Tuberculosis Control Programme (NTP) that was formulated by the National Tuberculosis Institute (NTI), Bangalore, based on some pioneering research done in India, served as a model for designing of tuberculosis programmes in many other countries. Halfdan Mahler, who later became the Director General of WHO and had worked as a researcher at NTI, said that many of the principles developed in the course of formation of the NTI directly fed into the Alma Ata declaration of 1978 (Mahler, 1985). However, these notable achievements also failed to deserve the support they needed from the government (Dujardin et al., 1997). In 1988, the Institute for Communications, Operations Research and Community Participation (ICORCI), which did a detailed study of the NTP provided 86 detailed recommendations to improve the functioning of NTP. It observed: 'It has been repeatedly brought to the attention of the Expert Team that NTP has been given a low priority. This has also been confirmed by the analysis of information collected' (ICORCI, 1988). Unfortunately, not even one of the ICORCI recommendations was acted upon by the government.

Primary Health Centres

The establishment of the first primary health centre (PHC) in October 1952 as part of the Community Development Programme (CDP) to provide integrated preventive, promotive and curative services was a landmark in the development of health care services in rural India. This was the first step towards implementation of the recommendations of the Bhore Committee (Dutt, 1965).

Social Orientation of Medical Education

In 1952, upgraded departments of preventive and social medicine were established in medical colleges to integrate the social, cultural and economic context of community health into the medical curriculum and provide a social dimension to the practice of clinical disciplines (Banerji, 1985).

Family Planning (Welfare) Programme

India was the first country to start a state-sponsored family planning programme in 1951 (First Plan period). Since then, the approaches of reducing population growth have taken various forms (Kishore, 2007).

The Mudaliar Committee (1962)

The Mudaliar Committee was set up in 1959 to review the progress made in the health sector during the first two plans and to lay down recommendations for the future. The Committee noted that even though mortality due to diseases such as malaria, smallpox, cholera, etc. had shown a substantial decline, basic health services had still not reached half the population. Not only was there a tremendous shortfall in the number of PHCs but the quality of services provided in them was very poor. Though doctors had been trained using public funds, they were actually doing private practice (Government of India, 1961). The gains of the vertical disease programmes were imperilled owing to deficiencies in the network of general health services such as the PHCs, which were supposed to have consolidated and maintained these gains (Batliwala, 1978). The condition of the secondary and district hospitals was no better, while curative services in the cities continued to grow.

The Mudaliar Committee recommended that there should be no further expansion in PHCs and efforts should be directed at consolidating them, thus bringing about a shift from 'coverage' to 'quality' of services. The overall thrust of the Committee was on the techno-centric approach to health care, emphasizing training more doctors, while the numbers of other medical personnel stagnated (Duggal, Undated). The context of socio-economic development seemed further detached from the scheme of improving the health of the people.

Other Committees

Several other committees were constituted from time to time to look into different aspects of health care services such as the problems of implementation of disease control programmes, multipurpose workers under the health and family planning programmes, health manpower planning and development, integration of health services and medical education (NIHFW, Undated).

Minimum Needs Programme

The lack of a meaningful impact of development during the 1950s and 60s on the lives of the poor in India led to the government developing a Minimum Needs Programme in the Fifth Five Year Plan. This programme was carried through to the Sixth Five Year Plan. It included elements of health, nutrition, water supply, environmental improvement, education, etc. (Centre for Policy Research, 1983).

The government came up with schemes to convert 'unipurpose' workers engaged in single disease programmes to multipurpose workers in 1971 (MoHFP, 1973) (and the Community Health Volunteers' scheme in 1977) (Bhattarcharji et al., 1986) in order to improve the delivery of basic health care to the people. However, these changes had minimal overall impact.

Primary Health Care

India committed itself to the WHO goal of 'Health for all by 2000 AD' in 1977 (WHO, 1981) and was a signatory to the resolution on provision of 'Comprehensive Primary Health Care (PHC)' as a strategy to reach the goal of 'Health for All' at the WHO Conference in Alma Ata in 1978 (WHO–UNICEF, 1978). However, these commitments have not translated to visible action and improvement in the health scenario.

Eradication of Smallpox

The eradication of smallpox comes through as a major achievement. The last case of smallpox occurred in India in May 1975 and WHO declared India a smallpox-free country in 1977.

National Health Policy (NHP) 1983

It was not till 1983 that the need for a health policy was recognized by our health planners. The NHP 1983 was a feeble attempt in the middle of the Sixth Plan period to synthesize recommendations of three important earlier committees—the Bhore Committee of 1946, the Mudaliar Committee and the Srivastava Committee (Singh and Singh, 2004). In the backdrop of 'Health for All by 2000 AD' and the Alma Ata declaration on primary health care, the NHP 1983 recommended 'universal, comprehensive primary health care services which are relevant to the actual needs and priorities of the community at a cost which people can afford' (Government of India, 1983). However, the policy failed to declare health care as a fundamental right of the people.

Five Year Plans

With respect to health, the Five Year plans have been high on rhetoric but have not been able to deliver on the ground. The die was cast from the First Plan when only 5.9% of the total plan outlay was committed to health as against a minimum of 15% recommended by the Bhore Committee. For the Second and Third Five Year Plans the outlay for health was 5% and 4.25%, respectively (Government of India, 1961).

After a series of lacklustre plans, the Sixth Plan stated that 'there is a serious dissatisfaction with the existing model of medical and health services with its emphasis on hospitals, specialization and super-specialization and highly trained doctors which is availed of mostly by the affluent classes. It is also realized that it is this model which is depriving the rural areas and the poor people of the benefits of good health and medical services' (Planning Commission, 1978). This plan was influenced by the Alma Ata declaration of Health for All by 2000 AD and the ICSSR–ICMR report of 1980 (ICSSR and ICMR, 1980). As a corrective measure the plan strategized provision of health services to the rural areas on a priority basis, training of a large cadre of first-level health workers selected from the community and emphasized that horizontal and vertical linkages had to be established among all inter-related programmes, such as water supply, environmental sanitation, hygiene, nutrition, education, family planning and maternal and child health (MCH) (Planning Commission, 1980) – an integrated approach at developing the health system and not just the health services system.

However, not only were no concrete plans drawn to implement the strategy of the Sixth Plan, but by the time of the Seventh Plan (1985–90) there was a discernible change in the tone, which set the stage for implementation of what is commonly referred to as 'Health Sector Reforms' (HSR). The Seventh Plan stated that 'our emphasis must be on greater efficiency, reduction of cost and improvement of quality. This calls for absorption of new technology, greater attention to economies of scale and greater competition' and 'development of specialized care and training in super-specialties would be encouraged in the public and the private sectors' (Planning Commission, 1985).

Beginning with a major economic crisis at the start of the Eighth Plan (1992–97), there has been a free fall through the Ninth (1997–02), Tenth (2002–07) and Eleventh Plan (2007–12) periods, in terms of what had been set out by the Bhore Committee. 'Health for All' got changed to 'Health for the Underprivileged' in the Eighth Plan (Planning Commission, 1992). Subsequently, the structural adjustment policies (SAP) and HSR were key elements as part of the philosophy of globalization, privatization and marketization of the health sector.

While the expenditure on communicable diseases decreased substantially from 28.4% of the layout for health in the Second Plan to 4.2% in the Eighth Plan, in the same period the expenditure on family planning increased from 1.3% to 26% of the layout for health (Table 1) (Qadeer, 2000). This was possibly a policy shift dictated by and reflecting the concern of international agencies and the Western world on population growth in developing countries (Planning Commission, 1992; Qadeer, 2000). However, socio-economic development is a necessary condition for population stabilization, as has happened in developed countries. The achievements of our population policy are a testament to this omission. Meanwhile, communicable diseases continue to claim many lives every year.

Table 1: Intrasectoral Financial Allocations for the Health Sector (in millions of Rupees)

Sub-Sector	*Five Year Plan*								
	First	*Second*	*Third*	*Annual*	*Fourth*	*Fifth*	*Sixth*	*Seventh*	*Eighth*
	1951–56	*1956–61*	*1961–66*	*1966–69*	*1969–74*	*1974–79*	*1980–85*	*1985–90*	*1992–97*
Control of communicable diseases	231 (16.5)	640 (28.4)	690 (27.7)	231 (10.2)	1270 (11.1)	2681.7 (11.5)	5240 (27)	10 126.7 (7.7)	10 450 (4.2)
Total health	903 (64.5)	1460 (64.9)	1500 (60.2)	939 (41.6)	4335 (37.5)	7962 (34.1)	18 211 (27)	33 928.9 (25.8)	75 759.5 (30.5)
Family planning	7 (0.5)	30 (1.3)	270 (10.8)	829 (36.7)	3150 (27.3)	5160 (22.1)	10 100 (15)	32 562 (24.7)	65 000 (26)
Water supply and sanitation	490 (35)	760 (35.8)	720 (28.9)	490 (21.7)	4070 (35.2)	10 220 (43.8)	39 220 (58)	55 970 (50.5)	107 430.3 (43)
Grand total (Health, family planning, water and sanitation)	1400	2250	2490	2258	15 555	23 342	57 530	131 716.5	248 189.8

Figures in parentheses are percentages of grand total, except for communicable diseases where the figures in parentheses are percentages of total health.
Source: Qadeer, 2000.

Structural Adjustment Programme and Health Sector Reforms

In the 1990s, we saw the implementation of what has been called the 'new economic policies' and 'structural adjustment' policies. Before being implemented in Asia, similar policies had been implemented in Latin America and Africa. These were a set of uniform strategies prescribed to countries by international funding agencies irrespective of the country's context and needs (World Bank, 1993).

The SAP led to the introduction of HSR in India. The main aspects of the International Monetary Fund–World Bank inspired reforms were: cuts in health sector investments, opening up of health care to the private sector, introduction of user fees, private investments in public hospitals, and techno-centric public health interventions (Qadeer, 2000). Cutbacks in the welfare sector resulted in a direct impact on primary health care (Qadeer, 2000). The poor have been the worst sufferers of these reforms. As three-fourths of the Indian population subsists on less than '20 a day' (Sen Gupta et al., 2007), access to health care is poor as 80 per cent of health care is in the private sector (Government of India, 2005) and health care in the public sector has had decreasing inputs over the past few decades. Nevertheless, health sector reforms have a strong constituency among the middle-and the upper middle-income groups who have largely opted for private health care services (Baru 1995; Iyer and Sen, 2000).

National Health Policy (NHP) 2002

The NHP 2002 is steeped in the spirit of free market economy and does away with socialistic policies in the health sector. The policy gives an important role to the private sector in the provisioning of health care. It says: 'The contribution of the private sector in providing health services would be much enhanced, particularly for the population group which can afford to pay for services... In principle, this policy welcomes the participation of the private sector in all areas of health activities—primary, secondary or tertiary... The policy also encourages the setting up of private insurance instruments for increasing the scope of coverage of the secondary and tertiary sector under private health insurance packages.' Even in respect of the poor the policy says: 'In the context of the very large number of poor in the country, it would be difficult to conceive of an exclusive government mechanism to provide health services to this category. It has sometimes been felt that a social health insurance scheme, funded by the government, and with service delivery through the private sector, would be the appropriate solution' (MoHFW, 2002).

As a result of this policy, a much larger and organized private health care system has evolved in the form of corporate hospitals, at the cost of large public subsidies, catering to the rich and health tourists, while large population groups in India do not have access to some of the most basic health care services.

National Rural Health Mission (NRHM)

The NRHM was launched in April 2005 in the backdrop of what has been described as the 'advanced stage of decay of the health services system, particularly the rural health service system of the country' by the Independent Commission on Health in India, set up under the aegis of the Voluntary Health Association of India (VHAI, 1997). Documents from the Planning Commission also paint an equally gloomy picture (Planning Commission, 1997 and 2003). The NRHM was an attempt to improve the provision of health care services to the rural people of India. However, the ability of NRHM to deliver on its stated objective has been seriously questioned by some leading public health experts since the time of its inception itself, given the manner of its conceptualization (Banerji, 2005).

The NRHM had envisaged increasing public spending on health from a meagre 0.9% of the gross domestic product in 2004–05 to up to 2%–3%. According to the National Health Accounts of the Ministry of Health and Family Welfare (MoHFW), it actually increased from 0.84% in 2004–05 to 1.1% in 2008–09, while the increase was from 1.19% to 1.45% in the economic survey 2009–10 (Planning Commission, 2003). An added problem is the inability of the states to use allocated funds at different levels of health care (Infochange Health, 2010; Government of India, 2009a). Poor allocation of funds translates into fewer resources for infrastructure development and poor infrastructure means lower utilization of even the meagre allocated funds. This leads to the argument that there is no point in increasing the budgetary allocation unless there is enhancement in the capacity of the states to use the funds.

The question remains as to how to optimize and use resources without changing a policy that supports private (for-profit) over public health care, curative over preventive and promotive health care, urban over rural health care and a medical education system that continues to train doctors who aspire for careers in urban, private sector hospitals and in developed countries rather than work in rural areas and among the poor and less privileged. Even where public funds are being spent, the emphasis is increasingly on public–private partnerships and the role of 'civil society organizations'. It is unclear how the conflicting aims of profit-oriented health care and publicly funded health care for the poor and needy will be reconciled in the public–private partnerships.

The Justice Qureshi Committee set up by the Delhi Government to look into the functioning of private hospitals in Delhi which had received large public grants in the form of free land and tax rebates, found that most of these hospitals had defaulted on their obligation towards treating poor patients free of cost (Qadeer and Reddy, 2006). The public component of the public–private partnerships can dominate only when public health care occupies an indisputable upper hand in overall health care—a stage that has been consigned to history in India.

The NRHM has resulted in progress in some states in terms of creating additional sub-centres, PHCs, community health centres, procurement of equipment and recruitment of personnel. However, there is lack of a comprehensive vision for improving the health system and thereby the health of the people. As on March 1, 2011 there were 45,062 doctors in the public sector to serve an estimated 833 million people in rural India, i.e. approximately one doctor to every 18,488 persons (presuming that all posts were occupied) (GOI, 2011).

The contradictions are glaring. The NRHM never envisaged the need to train in large numbers what Banerji has described as 'Managerial physicians, who have the epidemiological, managerial, social and political competence to provide leadership in the administration of the health services in the country' (Banerji, 2005). The important task of navigating the country's public health has instead been handed over to the 'generalist bureaucrats' or specialist clinicians sitting in the ministry who never had the opportunity to face the formidable challenges of rural health in India. Besides, health invariably is not a product only of efficient medical services. It is determined in the main by the social and economic condition of the people that determines their ability to earn, to eat, to afford a decent living and to access health care in need. Experts have estimated that rural poverty in India increased from 72% in 1973–74 to 87% in 2004–05 as per the original nutritional norms of per capita consumption of 2400 calories and 2100 calories for rural and urban India, respectively (Patnaik, 2007). India State Hunger Index Report published in 2009 calculated the hunger index for 17 Indian states. It states that 'not a single state in India falls in the low hunger or moderate hunger category defined by the Global Hunger Index 2008. Instead, most states fall in the alarming category, with Madhya Pradesh falling in the extremely alarming category. Four states—Punjab, Kerala, Andhra Pradesh and Assam—fall in the serious category. Punjab, which has the best hunger index score in India is placed below Gabon (in sub-Saharan Africa), Honduras and Vietnam' (Menon et al., 2009). However, there is not even a hint of how these pressing issues shall be tackled in NRHM, except of course some reference to intersectoral coordination.

Table 2: NRHM Goals for Reproductive and Child Health Indicators and Achievements by 2012

RCH II NRHM Indicator	RCH II NRHM Goal by 2012	Achievements by 2012
Maternal Mortality Ratio (MMR)	<100	178
Infant Mortality Rate (IMR)	< 30	42
Total Fertility Rate (TFR)	2.1	2.4

Source: The 2012 achievement figures for MMR, IMR and TFR have been obtained from Tables A. 56, A.41 and A.31 respectively of the Ministry of Health and Family Welfare (2013).

That NRHM was falling behind its objectives and targets had been evident even before the conclusion of seven years of its first phase in 2012. The Sixth Joint Review Mission Report of NRHM acknowledged that the Mission was way behind in achieving its targets set for various health indicators (GOI, 2009b). Table 2 gives the achievements of NRHM against the specific targets under 'reproductive and child health' set to be achieved by it. Available evidence suggests that the peaking of institutional deliveries, the core intervention implemented as part of NRHM to bring down the infant and maternal mortality, actually led to a remarkable slowing down of their rates of decline (Bajpai, 2014).

NRHM and Beyond

On May 15, 2013 the Government of India launched a 'National Urban Rural Mission' (NUHM) as a sub-mission under the overarching 'National Health Mission' that subsumed both NRHM and NUHM. NUHM was to be implemented in all cities and towns with more than fifty thousand population, district headquarters and state capitals (Government of India, 2013). The perfunctoral nature of the transition is evident from the fact that virtually the same pattern of organization of health services, as applicable for rural areas, was adopted for the urban areas as well, with some alteration in the population norms, without regard to the multiplicity of public authorities providing medical services in many of the cities, especially in large ones like the metros.

Meanwhile, even before there could be any serious reflection on the lessons to be drawn from implementation of NRHM, the idea of 'Universal Health Coverage' (UHC), as enunciated in the 'World Health Report, 2010' and passed by the 65th World Health Assembly in May 2012 at Geneva (Singh, 2013), firmly parked itself on the health policy agenda of the country.

The Planning Commission set up a High Level Expert Group (HLEG), with some noted public health figures/health activists in the country on the panel, to finalize the approach for implementation of 'UHC' in the country. The HLEG report, despite some of its eminent drawbacks, emphasized development and strengthening of the public health system for the delivery of UHC (Planning Commission, 2011). Its recommendations seemed like a breath of fresh air in an otherwise jarring health policy scenario; however even before these recommendations could make their way through, the HLEG was undermined and its recommendations debunked by the Planning Commission itself under pressure from the expected quarters. We shall dwell on this aspect in the next chapter.

The Planning Commission privileged report of its internal

'Steering Committee on Health set up to formulate the plan for the 12th Five Year Plan.' Summarizing the recommendations of the 'Steering Committee' the Jan Swasthya Abhiyan (People's Health Movement) stated:

> It is particularly problematic that the Plan document to be adopted by the panel by the end of this month, invokes the concept of Universal Health care, while it actually proposes a strategy that is far removed from the basic tenets of universal health care .... What is of greater concern is the strategy proposed for re-structuring of the country's health system in the document that proposes a transition from the present system which is a mix of public sector service provision plus insurance, to a system of health care delivered by a managed network. There, is thus, a road map envisaged where the government would abandon its central role of providing health care and become primarily just a manager of the new system (The Health Site, 2012).

The idea of 'insurance driven managed care' has been developed to a much greater extent in the 'Draft National Health Policy, 2015' (DNHP–2015) that was unveiled for public discussion by the Ministry for Health and Family Welfare in December 2014. We are not dwelling on this document over here as a separate chapter is being included in this volume on DNHP–2015. Nevertheless, the scheme laid out in DNHP–2015 only spells a death knell for publicly delivered health services in the country. The tragedy is that this may happen without the policy ever getting formally adopted, as public deception can work better by adhering to the unwritten policy paradigm.

With the coming of the Bharatiya Janata Party (BJP) led National Democratic Alliance (NDA) government at the centre, the mendacity wrecking the policy establishment has only got further accentuated. One of the reasons preventing the DNHP – 2015 from getting translated to official policy is said to be the displeasure it has incurred from the NITI (National Institution for Transforming India) Aayog—the Commission that has replaced the Planning Commission as the pinnacle of development policy formulation in the country.

Even the *'nominal'* reference to the strengthening of the public sector health care in the country has been objected to by the new planning body. We would like to quote the following passages from a letter written by the NITI Aayog to the MoHFW, which got leaked to the press (NITI Aayog, 2015), to bring home the point.

On increasing the health funding:

> There is universal agreement on the need for the government to step up expenditure on health, so in addition to an unambiguous commitment to increasing government spending on health, we also need to address ourselves to the question of how these additional resources will be deployed . . . . Also we need to assess whether drastically increasing investments will run into the law of diminishing marginal returns, besides posing a challenge to the absorptive capacities of the State Health Systems.

On its penchant for the private sector health care:

> While admitting that 80% outpatient and 60% inpatient care is provided by private health care providers as also the fact it is a $40 billion industry and that it is growing at a CAGR of 15%, the NHP document does not specifically indicate a framework for engaging these providers; barring expressing intent of regulating their quality through appropriate legislation or seeing it as a resource for filling critical gaps of the Public Sector. This to my mind is one of the principal weaknesses of the draft NHP document.

Hostility to the idea of free care

> Free care: A Chimera—The NHP aspires to create a health guaranteeing Assured Comprehensive Care , Free Drugs, Diagnostic, Emergency and Patient Transport Services to all in Public Health Facilities. This does not seem to be a reasonable supposition, given the budgetary and manpower constraints faced by the government system Predicating our strategy on such an assumption—when government has consistently struggled to provide even 1% of GDP to this structure in view of so many demands on the tax revenue—is an astounding leap of faith fraught with potentially unfortunate consequence that free services will be rationed as per budget/ manpower availability; the benefits of the subsidies being hogged by the rich and the connected and the poor to be left out on a limb or even worse being obligated to make informal payments to access the so called "free" services . At a time when the government is attempting to rationalize and better target the existing subsidy regime, it would be anachronistic to commit it to such an untargeted subsidy regime.

Conclusion

We have sketched above the trajectory of the development of the health services in India and it certainly is not the most desirable one. Have the governments since 1947 not been aware of these flaws? Governments could not possibly be as ignorant as that. There are nevertheless plausible reasons for the course of history of development of health services in India to have been what it has been post-1947. It is of utmost importance for every health worker seriously dedicated to the cause of improving the health of India's people to understand these reasons in order to place his or her efforts in perspective. In Chapter 4 we shall seek to understand some of these crucial factors that have shaped the development of health services in India.

REFERENCES

Banerji, D. (1985): *Health and Family Planning Services in India: An Epidemiological, Socio-Cultural and Political Analysis and a Perspective*, Lok Paksh, New Delhi, 23–26.

Batliwala, S. (1978): *The Historical Development of Health Services in India*, Foundation for Research in Community Health, Bombay.

Bhattarcharji, S., Abraham, S., Muliyil, J. et al. (1986): Evaluating Community Health Worker Performance in India, *Health Policy Plan*, Vol. 1: 232–9.

Baru, R.V. (1995): *Private Health care in India: Social Characteristics and Trends*. New Delhi: Sage Publications, 185.

Banerji, D. (2005): 'Politics of Rural Health in India.' *Indian Journal of Public Health*, Vol. 49 (3): 113-122. 34.

Bajpai, V. (2014): 'lmplementation of the Janani Sishu Suraksha Karyakram in Uttar Pradesh: Some Observations and Concerns,' *Indian Journal of Social Work*, October 2014; Vol. 75 (4): 573-594.

Centre for Policy Research (1983): *Population, Poverty and Hope*. Uppal Publishing House, New Delhi, 463–74.

Duggal, R. (Undated): *Health Planning in India*. Available from http://www.cehat.org/go/uploads/Publications/a168.pdf (accessed on November 29, 2015.

Dujardin, B., Kegels G., Buvé A. et. al. (1997): Tuberculosis Control: Did the Programme Fail or Did We Fail the Programme? *Tropical Medicine and International Health*, Vol. (2): 715–18.

Dutt, P.R. (1965): *Rural Health Services in India: Primary Health Centres*, 2nd edition, Central Health Education Bureau, New Delhi, 6.

Government of India (1946): *Report of the Health Survey and Development Committee:* The Bhore Committee Report, Vol. II, 1–17.

Government of India (1961): *Health Survey and Planning Committee (Mudaliar Committee)'*, Ministry of Health and Family Welfare, New Delhi.

Government of India (1983): *National Health Policy, 1983*, Ministry of Health and Family Welfare, New Delhi.

Government of India (2005): *'Current Status of the Private Sector in India'* in the *'Executive Summary, Report of the National Commission on Macroeconomics and Health.'* New Delhi: Ministry of Health and Family Welfare, 5.

Government of India (2009a): *National Rural Health Mission. Third Common Review Mission Report, January 15 to February 8, 2007.* New Delhi: Ministry of Health and Family Welfare, 48–49, 69–70, 111.

Government of India (2011): *Bulletin of Rural Health Statistics in India.* New Delhi: Ministry of Health and Family Welfare, Tables 21, 28 and 28A.

Government of India (2009b): *National Rural Health Mission. Sixth Joint Review Mission, May 25 to July 7, 2009.* New Delhi: Ministry of Health and Family Welfare.

Government of India (2013): 'Resolution on National Urban Health Mission', Resolution No. L.19017/1/2008-UH (Vol. III) dated May 15, 2013, Ministry of Health and Family Welfare, New Delhi.

Harrison, M. (1994): *Public Health in British India: Anglo-Indian Preventive Medicine, 1859–1914,* Cambridge University Press, Cambridge and New York.

ICORCI (Institute of Communication, Operations Research and Community Involvement) (1988): *In Depth Study on National Tuberculosis Programme of India*, Koramangala, Bangalore, November.

Indian Council of Social Science Research (ICSSR) and Indian Council of Medical Research (ICMR) (1980): *'Health for All: An Alternative Strategy'*, Report of the Joint Study Group, Indian Institute of Education (Publisher), Pune.

Iyer, A., Sen G. (2000): *Health Sector Changes and Health Equity in the 1990s in India.* In: Raghuram, S. (ed). *Health and Equity–Effecting Change,* Technical Report Series 1.8, HIVOS, 2000:15–55.

Infochange Health (2010): *NRHM Completes Five Years.* Available at http://infochangeindia.org/201004138231/Health/News/NRHM-completes-fiveyears.html (accessed on May 22, 2010).

Jain, A. (2012): Current Status of Leprosy as Seen in a Tertiary Care Hospital in North India. *Journal of Medical Researh*, Vol. 135 (3): 439–40.

Kishore, J. (2007): *National Health Programmes of India,* 7th editon, New Century Publications, New Delhi, 93–197.

Mushtaq, M.U. (2009): Public Health in British India: A Brief Account of the History of Medical Services and Disease Prevention in Colonial India. *Indian Journal of Community Medicine*, Vol. 34 (1): 6–14.

Madras Public Health Act (1939): Available from http://www.sanchitha.ikm.in/sites/default/files/MadrasPublicHealth_ %20Act1939.pdf (Accessed on November 29, 2015).

Mehta, B., Nayak, C., Savant, S. et al. (2009): Leprosy in the era of integration, *Indian Journal of Dermatol Venereol Leprol*, Vol. 75:190–1.

Mahler, H. (1985): 'Address at National Tuberculosis Institute' In *'Proceedings of Silver Jubilee Celebrations'*, National Tuberculosis Institute, Bangalore, 82.

MoHFP (Ministry of Health and Family Planning) (1973): *Report of the Committee on Multipurpose Workers Under Health and Family Planning Programme*, Government of India, New Delhi.

Ministry of Health and Family Welfare (MoHFW) (2002): *National Health Policy-2002*, Government of India, New Delhi.

Menon, P., Deolalikar A., Bhaskar A. (2009): *India State Hunger Index: Comparisons of Hunger Across States.* Washington DC, Bonn, and Riverside: International Food Policy Research Institute, Welthungerhilfe and University of California.

Ministry of Health and Family Welfare (2013): *Health and Family Welfare Statistics of India, 2013*, Government of India, October.

Nelson, D. (2012): Leprosy on the Rise in India Seven Years After Disease was 'Eradicated', *The Telegraph*, September 19. Available at http:// www.telegraph.co.uk/news/worldnews/ asia/india/9552979/ Leprosy-on-the-rise-in-India-seven-years-after-disease-was-eradicated.html (accessed on January 1, 2013).

NIHFW (National Institute of Health and Family Welfare) (Undated): *'National Health Committees'*. Available at http://nihfw.org/NDC/ DocumentationServices/Committe_and_ commission.html (accessed on September 23, 2009). NITI Aayog (2015): Letter No. 4 (6)/2 0 15-H&FW dated August 10, 2015 addressed to the 'Economic Advisor' in the MoH&FW regarding revised comments on draft NHP 2015.

Planning Commission (1978): *Draft Sixth Five Year Plan*, Vol. III, Government of India, New Delhi, p. 250.

Planning Commission (1980): Chapter 22 on *'Health, Family Planning and Nutrition' in 'Sixth Five Year Plan, 1980–85' Document*, Government of India, New Delhi. Available at http://planningcommission.nic.in/ plans/planrel/fiveyr/6th/ 6planch22.html (accessed on May 23, 2010).

Planning Commission (1985): 'Foreword' in *'Seventh Five Year Plan' Document*, Government of India, New Delhi. Available at http:// planningcommission. nic.in/plans/planrel/fiveyr/7th/vol1/ 7v1fore.htm (accessed on May 23, 2010).

Planning Commission (1992): 'Objectives and Orientation' in the *'Eighth Five Year Plan' Document*, Government of India, New Delhi. Available at *h*ttp:// planningcommission.nic.in/plans/planrel/fiveyr/8th/ vol1/8ch1.htm (accessed on May 23, 2010).

Planning Commission (1997): *Ninth Five Year Plan (1997–2002).* Planning Commission, Government of India, New Delhi.

Planning Commission (2003): *Tenth Five Year Plan (2002–2007).* Planning

Commission, Government of India, New Delhi.

Patnaik, U. (2007): Neoliberalism and Rural Poverty in India, *Economic and Political Weekly* 2007; 42: 3132–50.

Planning Commission (2011): Report of the 'High Level Expert Group Report on Universal Health Coverage for India', November.

Qadeer, I. (2000): Health care Systems in Transition III. India, Part I. The Indian Experience, *Journal Public Health Medicine*, Vol. 22: 25–32.

Qadeer I., Reddy S. (2006): Medical Care in the Shadow of Public Private Partnership, *Social Scientist* 2006; 34: 4–20.

Sokhey Committee Report (1948): *National Planning Committee Series: Report of the Sub-Committee on National Health*, Vora and Co (Publishers), Bombay, 12.

Singh, A.R., Singh, S.A. (2004): *The Goal: Health For All, The Commitment: All for Health.* Mens Sana Monographs 2004, 2: 97–110.

Sen Gupta, A., Kannan, K.P., Srivastava, R.S. et al. (2007): *'Report on Conditions of Work and Promotion of Livelihoods in the Unorganized Sector'*, National Commission for Enterprises in the Unorganized Sector, Government of India.

Singh Zile (2013): 'Universal Health Coverage for India by 2022: A Utopia or Reality?' *Indian Journal of Community Medicine*, April-June, Vol. 38(2): 70–73.

TheHealthSite.Com (2012): 'Health care Activists Balk at 12th Five Year Plan Document's Proposals.' Available from http://www.thehealthsite.com/news/health care-activists-balk-at-12th-five-year-plan-documents-proposals/ on December 14, 2015.

Voluntary Health Association of India (VHAI) (1997): *Report of the 'Independent Commission on Health in India.'* New Delhi.

World Health Organization (WHO) (1981): *Global Strategy for Health for All by the Year 2000*, Geneva.

WHO–UNICEF (1978): *Primary Health Care: Report of the International Conference on Primary Health Care, Alma-Ata, USSR.* Health for all Series No 1, September 6–12, Geneva, WHO.

World Bank (1993): *World Development Report 1993: Investing in Health.* Oxford: Oxford University Press.

4

Factors That Influenced the Development of Health Services in India*

Chapter Three traced the development of modern health care services in India from colonial times up to the launch of the National Rural Health Mission and the most recent policy initiatives. The analysis emphasizes that this development is guided by various national and international contradictions between social classes and countries. This chapter explores how exactly these contradictions shaped the development of health services in India.

Class Contradictions within Indian Society and Their Influence on the Health Services

The development paradigm pursued by India's ruling élite since 1947 has been structured primarily to serve their interests and those of the sections of society whose support is crucial to maintain their grip on power while the impoverished majority has had to remain content with minor concessions. In India, while on one hand we have a minuscule class that is extremely rich and has maintained a pervasive control over the country's resources and to whom the British bequeathed political power in 1947, on the other is the vast multitude (nearly 77 per cent of the population) of people who struggle to eke out an existence on a per capita daily consumption

---

* This chapter had initially been published as an article in the *National Medical Journal of India* and is being reproduced here with some modifications with the permission of the journal. The full reference of the earlier article is – Bajpai, Vikas, Anoop Saraya (2014): Factors that Influenced the Development of Health Services in India. *NMJI*, Vol. 25 (4): 240-244.

of up to Rs. 20 a day (GOI, 2007). Sandwiched in between is a middle class of approximately 50 million Indians (Ablet et. al., 2007) with dreams of making it to the big league, and to that extent serving as a bulwark of the ruling élite.

India's ruling classes have been nurtured to imbibe a colonial mindset and a way of life and thinking akin to their erstwhile colonial masters. It is instructive here to recall Thomas Macaulay's famous Minute of February 2, 1835 on education in India. Addressing the British Parliament he said: 'We must at present do our best to form a class who may be interpreters between us and the millions whom we govern; a class of persons, Indian in blood and colour, but English in taste, in opinions, in morals, and in intellect" (Macaulay, 1835).

History provides ample testimony of the British having succeeded in that endeavour. This inevitable conclusion is amply borne out by the mores of the Indian élite. The former Prime Minister, Dr. Manmohan Singh, said at Oxford:

> Today, with the balance and perspective offered by the passage of time and the benefit of hindsight, it is possible for an Indian Prime Minister to assert that India's experience with Britain had its beneficial consequences too. Our notions of the rule of law, of a constitutional government, of a free press, of a professional civil service, of modern universities and research laboratories have all been fashioned in the crucible where an age-old civilization met the dominant Empire of the day. These are all elements which we still value and cherish. Our judiciary, our legal system, our bureaucracy, and our police are all great institutions, derived from British-Indian administration and they have served the country well (Singh, 2005).

That there was barely a murmur of protest from any section of the ruling élite to such unabashed glorification of colonial rule by an Indian prime minister underlines their agreement with this view.

This indeed, raises the question of whether Indians were so incapable of giving themselves the 'rule of law', 'universities for higher education', 'a constitution', 'a free press', and an 'efficient bureaucracy', that they needed the benevolent crutch of the 'British Empire'. Could anyone be closer to eulogizing the great 'civilizing mission' of the 'white man'?

Indian independence in 1947 was nothing more than a transfer of power (Hansard, 1947 a) brought about by an act of the British Parliament (Hansard, 1947 b). Unlike the case of China, where the revolution of 1949 entailed radical socio-economic and political restructuring of the society, 'Indian Independence' ensured a continuance of the old social, economic and political order. Take, for example, the case of the Indian Civil Service. The Indian Civil Service (ICS) under the British did more than just administer India: it represented the Raj and was charged with securing its dominance (Burra, 2007). ICS officers often described themselves as 'rulers' rather than 'servants' (Woodruff, 1959; Gilmour, 2007). However, these very ICS officers who in the perception of the Indian masses were 'neither Indian, nor civil, nor servants' continued to rule even after the transfer of power. This only ensured a continuance of policies seeped in a colonial mindset.

The medical profession is in a sense owned by and forms one segment of the élite section of Indian society. It shares a mutuality of interest with the political, bureaucratic, business, and the feudal classes given their common class origins. It is no surprise then that the urban, educated governing élite have fostered health policies that have led to the development of highly techno-centric, predominantly curative health care services concentrated in the cities. The interests of the medical profession are best served by the development of highly profitable curative health care that ensures their élite status in the society. There is enormous pressure from within the profession as well as from the medical technology industry for the government to establish highly specialized services in the urban centres. These services are exorbitantly expensive to maintain, let alone to establish, and are inevitably available to only a minuscule segment of the population (Zurbrigg, 1991).

Prioritization of the health needs of the common people potentially calls into question all the national policy initiatives adopted and the privileges that have accrued through continuing iniquitous distribution of land, industrial resources, and the dual education policy adopted that has enabled professional education to be monopolized by the rich. What is essential is a complete overhaul of the entire system of education and health care, which is unlikely to occur because it militates against the interests of the constituencies of those in power. An attempt to restructure health care is to order the restructuring of the society itself– something, that is worse than nemesis for the ruling classes (Ibid., 107).

The Development Paradigm in the Immediate Post-Independence Period and Its Impact on the Development of the Health Services

At the time of independence in 1947, India was a backward economy. Given its poor technological and scientific capabilities, industrialization was limited and lopsided. The agricultural sector retained features of feudal and semi-feudal institutions, resulting in low productivity. The means of transport and communications were underdeveloped, educational and health facilities were inadequate, and social security measures virtually non-existent. In brief, poverty was rampant and unemployment widespread, resulting in a generally low standard of living (Prasad, 2007).

At this stage there were two models open to India to follow. That of a planned socialist economy as in the Soviet Union, a country that had been among the most backward countries of Europe till the October Revolution, but built its economy singlehandedly by placing reliance on its own resources in face of international isolation from the developed countries of the West. The second option was adopting the economic models of development that had gained currency in the post-war West.

Following an outright capitalist path of development was not feasible for a country such as India. The big Indian bourgeoisie, even though fattened by huge profits from wartime contracts (Chibber, 2003), still lacked the kind of capital required for investment in the development of heavy industries and infrastructure to build a base for India's economic development. A plan for the economic growth of India, known as the 'Bombay Plan', was proposed by seven leading Indian industrialists for the economic development of India, which appeared in two volumes in 1944 and 1945 (Thakurdas, 1945). The plan proposed that, "in the event that the private sector could not immediately do so—the establishment of critical industries as public sector enterprises while simultaneously ensuring a market for the output through planned purchases by the government" (Anstey, 1945).

On the other hand, the Keynesian economic model, which propagated a predominant private sector, but with a large role of government and the public sector for macroeconomic stability (Sullivan and Sheffrin, 2003), was gaining currency in the Anglo-American world as a means of reconstructing the war-ravaged economies of the West (Hazlitt, 1959). Added to this was the notion that the capitalism supported by the state would have a trickle-down effect, thereby also benefiting those lower down the economic ladder. The mixed economic model which India adopted was based on Keynesian principles (Backhouse, 2002).

Simultaneously the United Nations Monetary and Financial Conference, commonly known as the Bretton Woods Conference was organized in July 1944 to regulate the international monetary and financial order after the conclusion of the Second World War (Markwell, 2006). This conference gave rise to the Bretten Woods institutions—the International Monetary Fund and International Bank for Reconstruction and Development (IBRD), later known as the World Bank. Even though the purpose of IBRD's creation was to speed up post-war reconstruction and aid political stability, the seminal idea of the Bretten Woods Conference was the notion of open markets. India was a participatory member country in the conference (IMF Archives, Undated).

It must also be understood here that there was an understanding in the world and amongst the developing countries, that it was not necessary for them to adopt the tortuous process of socio-political and economic development experienced by countries in the West in order to ensure their development; all they needed to do was to ape the model as established in the developed countries of the West. India's ruling classes thus embarked on a path which has been described as 'state-led capitalism' (Kelkar, 2005), following in the footsteps of the economic pattern being adopted in the West. The state became the entrepreneur and considerable physical infrastructure, heavy industries, and knowledge institutions were created. However, minimal effort was devoted to developing agriculture and abolishing its semi-feudal relations of production. There was some land reform legislation albeit half-hearted and ineffective. Given the backwardness of agriculture, the overwhelming majority of the people dependent on it for their livelihood continued to remain impoverished, thus limiting the growth of markets for India's expanding industrial base. Continued economic backwardness resulted in a lack of genuine political empowerment of the people at large and thus an effective say in the policy matters, including the development of the health services. Drawing its lineage from an international policy framework dominated by the West, the development path chosen by India provided a stable base for the continuing domination of Western interests of its social, economic, and political development, a process described as neo-imperialism.

It was this development paradigm that influenced the development of health care services in independent India. It is instructive here to recall the words of Debabar Banerji:

> Each pattern of approach to health care emerges as a logical outcome of a given political, social and economic system. These forces generate an unwritten policy frame which influences the health of a population (Banerji, 2008).

A mixed economy saw the public sector lead health service development together with a significant involvement of the private sector. Urban areas received over three-fourths of the medical care resources while rural areas had to remain content with 'special attention' under the Community Development Programme (CDP) (Duggal, 2002). The vertical disease control programmes launched immediately after independence with financial assistance and technical guidance from Western agencies subscribed to the belief that diseases could be controlled by combating the spread of germs through modern technological interventions. This orientation ignored the social determinants of disease such as inadequate nutrition, clothing, and housing, and the lack of sanitary conditions. The national malaria eradication programme (NMEP) was started in 1953 with aid from the Technical Cooperation Mission of the USA and the technical advice of the WHO. In the initial TB control programme emphasis was given to BCG vaccination. These programmes depended on international agencies like the UNICEF, WHO, and the Rockefeller Foundation for supplies of necessary pesticides and vaccines. Along with financial aid came political and ideological influence. The experts of various international agencies decided the entire policy framework, programme design, financial commitments, etc. (Duggal, 2002).

These policies did not however have the anticipated effect. The continuing lack of access of the majority to quality medical care, two decades after independence led to questions being raised regarding the choices made at the time of Independence. A number of subsequent official committees diagnosed this to be the consequence of an 'urban-oriented, curative, technology centred evolution of health services alienated from the masses.' The fact that the policy planners were time and again compelled to at least talk about reorienting this development is evidence of the primary tension that continues to challenge the élitist orientation of health care (Ritu Priya, 2005).

Period of the 1970s and 80s and Primary Health care

The golden age of capitalism, spanning a period in the mid-20th century from 1950 to 1973 came to an end with the oil crisis of the 1970s. The decision of the Arab members of the Organization of Petroleum Exporting Countries (OPEC) to impose an oil embargo in response to the decision of the US government to resume military supplies to Israel during the Yom Kippur war led to a steep hike in the global prices of oil leading to an 'oil price shock' together with the 1973-4 stock market crash (Perron, 1988). Because of their dependence on oil as the principal source of energy, the major capitalist economies, and principally those of the US, UK, Canada, Japan, and Netherlands entered a period of prolonged stagnation and high inflation due to industrial slowdown, shortage of production, and the high prices of goods (DeLong, 1998; Burda and Wyplosz, 1997; Hall and Taylor, 1988).

Simultaneously two other events of extreme importance in world history occurred which had a profound impact on world politics: the defeat of the US in the Vietnam War in 1975 (Wikipedia, undated) and the entry of the People's Republic of China into the United Nations in 1971 (UPI.com, 1971). Subsequently, the People's Republic of China gained membership of the WHO.

The economic recession in the leading capitalist economies followed by these two events led to a loss of the capitalist sheen and in particular a tremendous loss of face for US imperialism. The 'golden age of capitalism' notwithstanding, the economic disparities between the haves and the have-nots had persisted even in the Western world (Gindin, 2002; Huges and Fergusson, 2000).[2]

The much touted 'trickle down' economics had produced a massive flood-up. The entire decade of the 1960s and 70s was characterized worldwide by massive people's movements: students' movements in Europe and the US, an anti-war movement and a civil rights movement in the US, the establishment of socialism in Cuba after the revolution in 1959, the Naxalbari movement and the political turbulence in India leading to the imposition of emergency and the Cultural Revolution in China. This had a sobering effect on governments across the world and forced them to make concessions to the underclass, including concessions for a more pro-people health care system. The entry of China into the WHO compelled the world to take note of the impressive gains that the country had made in improving the health of its people as a whole through the 'barefoot' doctors model and their innovative experiments in low cost health care during the Cultural Revolution (Daquing and Unschuld, 2008).

It was against the background of these conditions obtaining in the decade of the 1970s, that the goal of 'Health For All by 2000 AD' was adopted by the 30th World Health Assembly in 1977 at the Alma Ata Conference (WHO, 1981). This committed countries across the world that health should not be considered merely a technical question but one that should be at the very centre of the social, economic, and political planning of countries. Above all, it was recognized that providing 'Health For All' was a political question. Health became a right of the people wherein achieving the highest possible level of health and not just the bare minimum was considered necessary for the development of the people. From the realm of theory, the goal of 'Health For All' was sought to be put in practice and 'Primary Health Care' was placed at the centre of a new 'bottom-up' strategy to achieve it as opposed to the earlier 'top-down' approach of the top-heavy 'curative model' of health-care. Health was no longer to be the concern of individuals but the prime concern of society as a whole (WHO and UNICEF, 1978 a).

It is an altogether different matter that most of the governments reneged on implementing 'Primary Health Care' almost as soon as they committed themselves to it. That, however, is not a failure of the idea but remains a failure of the ruling classes across the world, and certainly not the least in India. The idea continues to resonate in the hearts and minds of all thinking and caring people.

Undoing of Alma Ata and Thereafter

The entrenched interests of those in the medical industry (pharmaceutical, medical appliances, medical insurance, private for profit health care) and the political class nurtured by them felt threatened by the very idea of primary health care and rightly so for it was anticipated that the 'proper application of primary health care will have far-reaching consequences, not only throughout the health sector but also for other social and economic sectors at the community level. Moreover, it will greatly influence community organization in general. Resistance to such change is only to be expected...." (WHO and UNICEF, 1978 b).

Health ministries in developing countries, prompted by international funding agencies and consultants, began to launch national programmes based on primary health care. In practice however it was a continuation of the same top-down approach. To sustain the new image, the progressive language of Alma Ata was co-opted: catch phrases such as 'people's participation', 'decision-making by the people', and 'empowerment' became part of the new official jargon (David and David, 1997).

'Central control, however, remained intact. While community participation was encouraged, it was generally the participation of weak compliance, rather than the strong participation of decision-making control. Community health workers (CHWs) were trained, but rather than being the most important members of the health team, they were relegated to the lowest, most subservient position in the existing health hierarchy' (David and David, 1997). This mirrors the all too familiar story of trial and error by our own health policy-makers in India.

The Coup D'état at Bellagio and Selective Primary Health care

Concerned about the identification of the most cost-effective health strategies, the Rockefeller Foundation sponsored in 1979 a small conference on Health and Population in Development at its Bellagio Conference Centre in Italy. The goal of the conference was to examine the status and interrelations of health and population programmes as the organizers detected 'disturbing signs of declining interest in population issues' (Kanagaratnam, 1979). The heads of important agencies were involved in the organization of the conference: Robert S. McNamara, former secretary of defence in the Kennedy and Johnson administrations and, since 1968, President of the World Bank; Maurice Strong, chairman of the Canadian International Development and Research Centre; David Bell, vice president of the Ford Foundation; and John J. Gillian, administrator of the US Agency for International Development, among others, were involved (Cueto, 2004). So as it happened, all the real big bosses of the international policy establishment were all present.

The conference was based on a published paper by Julia Walsh and Kenneth S. Warren entitled 'Selective Primary Health Care: An Interim Strategy for Disease Control in Developing Countries' (Walsh and Warren, 1979). The paper sought to identify the specific causes of death, paying special attention to the most common diseases afflicting infants in developing countries such as diarrhoea and diseases that stemmed from lack of immunization. The authors did not openly criticize the Alma-Ata Declaration. They presented an 'interim' strategy or entry points through which basic health services could be developed. They also emphasized 'attainable goals' and " 'cost-effective' planning. In the paper, and at the meeting, selective primary health care was introduced as the name of a new perspective. To put it mildly, the terms 'attainable goals' and 'cost-effective' implied practicality: don't be sentimental about people's health, for the world is a real place not an ideal one. While 'primary health care' may be good it is not entirely feasible. Primary Health Care was thus substituted by Selective Primary Health Care and the two concepts were worlds apart The opportunity for the development of self-reliant development of health systems in the developing countries that was offered by the 'Primary Health Care' approach was thus lost to 'selective primary health care'.

Reaganomics and Thatcherite Conservatism and Their Impact on Health

Almost a decade long recession and inflation in the major economies in the Anglo-American world led to a disillusionment with Keynesian economics. In the sphere of economics the counter revolution was led by free market economist Milton Friedman of Chicago School fame, whereby the 'altruistic pretensions' of the state came under increasing attack (Backhouse, 2002). In the realm of politics it led to the resurgence of the right. In the UK, Margaret Thatcher of the Conservative Party came to power in 1979 and led the charge to help 'topple the welfare state and make the world safer for capitalism' (Johnson, 1998). In the US it was Reaganomics that fully displaced Keynesianism in 1981 with the election of Ronald Reagan as president. The displacement of Keynesianism was a gradual process that began with the implementation of monetary policies to control the inflation that was spiralling and then gradually being transformed into a 'silent revolution' displacing development economics with free market tendencies by the mid-1980s (Green, 2003). In the South Americas the efforts at displacing development economics were far more visible: for instance, the 1973 coup by Augusto Pinochet in Chile and other military dictatorships, which brought in governments strongly favouring free market economies (Henales and Edwards, 2002). In the developing countries of Africa and Asia the commitment to development economics largely faded away and by the mid-1980s the free market agenda was broadly accepted (Boughton, 2001). Even in the erstwhile socialist China, the Deng Xiaoping leadership launched in 1978 pro-market reforms under the garb of 'Socialism with Chinese Characteristics' (Hu, 2005). These developments set the tone for a gradual jettisoning of the 'Socialist rhetoric' in India, which had hitherto served as an effective cloak for an otherwise private capital-friendly orientation of the economy.

Impact of These Developments on the Health Services

We have traced through the article how the policy orientation of the Indian health establishment had dovetailed that of their role models in the West with the utmost fidelity. The national and international developments sketched out in this section were no exception to this phenomenon. The withdrawal of the state virtually all over the world from the sphere of social welfare was epitomized in Reagan's inaugural speech: 'Government is not the solution to our problem, government is the problem' (Reagan, 1981). Ronald Reagan's views opposing 'Socialized Medicine' had been known since 1961 when he 'criticized Social Security for *supplanting* private savings and warned that subsidized medicine would curtail Americans' freedom' and that 'pretty soon your son won't decide when he's in school, where he will go or what he will do for a living. He will wait for the government to tell him' (Lowenstein, 2009). Thatcher on her part made a spirited attempt to dismantle the National Health Service in the UK (BBC, 1999). The cynicism of the Thatcher era is reflected in her statement given to the magazine *Woman's Own*: 'There is no such thing as society. There are individual men and women, and there are families. And no government can do anything except through people, and people must look after themselves first. It is our duty to look after ourselves and then to look after our neighbour' (Thatcher, 1987). This obviates any responsibility whatsoever on the part of the government towards people's health.

These developments were mirrored in the health policy in India. The involvement of the Indian state in caring for the health of its people, which at no point was comprehensive, began becoming even more lethargic. By the 1980s private health care in India had begun acquiring a dominant role for itself. Data in the 1980s from micro-studies and national level studies by the National Sample Survey and the National Council of Applied Economic Research (NCAER) provided the necessary evidence to show the overwhelming dominance of the private health sector in India (Duggal, 1998). Additionally, as we shall see later, the World Bank came to have an increasing say in India's health policies, as indeed those of other developing countries.

The Balance of Payment Crisis in Developing Countries in the 1980s and its Impact on Health

The debt crisis in the developing countries, which reached a peak in 1982, actually had its genesis in the mid-1970s. The oil crises of 1973 stemming from the Arab-Israeli war, and that of 1979 in the wake of the Iranian revolution, came as a financial windfall for petroleum exporting countries in terms of the income from spiralling prices resulting in a massive build up of surplus capital by the OPEC countries which was deposited in Western Banks. Now banks wouldn't keep money for nothing, so OECD countries actively encouraged the recycling of this built up capital through extension of loans to developing countries on very liberal terms, and often without adequate credit analysis (Akanle, 1992).

In face of the ongoing stagflation and political reasons, the aid from the West to the developing countries dried up, thus creating an imperative for increased borrowing from the Western banks flush with cash. This borrowing spree in most cases led to the purchase of consumer items, obsolete equipment and machinery in keeping with the premise of aping the West to develop yourselves, or for projects that never took off or later became 'white elephants' (Akanle, 1992). A pertinent case in point is the aid extended by the UK government subject conditional on India purchasing helicopters from the UK Westland Company which was facing closure for lack of demand. Almost immediately after these purchases were made, Indian lives were lost in accidents involving these helicopters and the helicopters were declared unfit for use (Bagchi, undated).

There was a gradual build-up in the external debt of Third World countries from the 1970s till it reached unmanageable proportions in the early 1980s. Simultaneously, there was a drop in the international prices of primary commodities (cash crops like cotton and mineral ores) which constituted the primary exports of the Third World countries, which further worsened the debt crisis (Akanle, 1992). High levels of corruption, political instability in many developing countries, and lack of governmental managerial expertise are some of the other factors which compounded the situation. The balance of payment crisis reached a point where the countries concerned were obliged to take further loans from multilateral agencies for servicing the interest on loans. These loans came with strings attached, having wide-ranging consequences for the sovereignty of the countries and the welfare of their people.

Bretten Woods: Conditionalities and Consequences for Health

It is now widely acknowledged that the Structural Adjustment Programme (SAP) implemented as a part of the New Economic Policies in the various Third World countries came as a necessary condition of the loans extended by the World Bank and the IMF to them, especially since 1980. Many of us have had the lived experience of the current phase of the SAP on health care in India since its inception in 1991 with the unleashing of the era of globalization, either as health care professionals, as consumers of health care in various forms, as concerned citizens keen to understand the impact of these policies on our people or as activists opposed to their implementation. Suffice it is here to bring home the essence of these policies which have unquestionably led to the growth of market-oriented health care services.

As we have discussed above, not only has the spirit of these so-called New Economic Policies been an essential part of our development paradigm since the time of 'transfer of power' to India's ruling classes in 1947, but that the structural reforms actually began much earlier than is commonly believed. India had embarked upon the process of substantive reforms in economic policies in the early 1980s when it decided to approach the IMF for a loan of over $ 5 billion (the largest loan given by the Fund till then) by accepting conditions which were widely believed to have compromised India's sovereignty (Chaudhary et al., 2004). A regimen of fiscal prudence in the form of a Structural Adjustment Programme (SAP) was unleashed with full force.

The essence of SAP was the conversion of the erstwhile 'market economies' to 'market societies'. In the words of John Gray, Oxford Professor of Political Science and a staunch Thatcherite, the difference between the two is that, while in 'market economies' 'markets are embedded within the broader social relations and, in part, constrained by them'; in 'market societies' ,'society is made to run as if it is more or less an adjunct to the market'. The implication of this for health planning is that while in 'market societies' it might still be possible for the private health sector to share social concerns for the health of the people apart from the profit garnered, in a market society the unabashed use of health-care for the pursuit of profit becomes an exalted virtue. Even public sector health care does not remain untouched by this. Market principles such as revenue generation, monetary incentives for the doctors and paramedical staff have today become the accepted norms in public sector health care. Worse still, it is projected that people will work only under two conditions: either for monetary incentives or for fear of losing them; no one it appears will work because the creation of a better society is an essential human trait, an idea that is very problematic. There is apparently little desire to look at the system that neither provides the conditions where an individual's work becomes his overriding virtue, nor acknowledges the work of the selfless millions in the country.

The results of such an orientation are self-evident. A qualitative study into the 'Subaltern Health Care Consumption Under Neoliberalism' in India, undertaken in a large city, Kanpur, gives us a glimpse of the reality on the ground. Here, the largest state-owned hospital in the city, traditionally an important source of health care for subaltern groups, notwithstanding its excellent infrastructure, was completely marred by the apathy of its physicians and support staff and their utter negligence to the needs of their subaltern consumers. Patients repeatedly complained that the physicians and paramedical staff did not provide proper care to the subaltern groups because of their low financial capacity (Varman and Ram Manohar, 2007). The poignancy of the situation is driven home by the following field notes mentioned in the study:

> The (general) ward was full of patients lying on beds in the room. On the last bed of this ward a woman was lying with her face covered. She appeared to be very thin and there was no perceivable movement of the chest. The slow moving fan blew a portion of her sari . . . the arm got exposed with multiple needle marks and dried blood stains. The stains of blood and plasma appeared to be fresh. The patient on the bed next to her informed me that she was dead (Varman and Ram Manohar, 2007).

Belated Course Correction

The dark side of 'globalization' and 'structural reforms' in terms of human development has become too obvious to be ignored either nationally or internationally. Gradually but steadily, the virtues of the 'welfare state' are being reinvented to lend globalization a human face. Paul Krugman, the American economist awarded the Nobel Prize for economics in 2008 cites Gregory Mankiw to say this of Keynes against the backdrop of the economic meltdown in 2008:

> If you were going to turn to only one economist to understand the

> problems facing the economy, there is little doubt that the economist would be John Maynard Keynes. Although Keynes died more than a half-century ago, his diagnosis of recessions and depressions remains the foundation of modern macroeconomics. His insights go a long way towards explaining the challenges we now confront (Krugman, 2008).

Krugman is not alone in remembering Keynes. Prior to him have been Joseph Stiglitz (Nobel Prize laureate and former chief economist of the World Bank) and our own Amartya Kumar Sen, who have begun singing paeans to state intervention in the economy to safeguard public good. Having rocked a gaping hole at the base of the world economy, the world's biggest bankers sought state bailouts to save them. The very system needs to be bailed out, and therefore the need to eulogize Keynesianism through Nobel for the Krugmans, Stiglitzs, and Sens of the world.

Alerted by the bombed 'Shining India' campaign of the NDA government, the United Progressive Alliance (UPA) I government led by the Congress came up with programmes such as the National Rural Health Mission (NRHM), the Mahatma Gandhi National Rural Employment Guarantee Scheme (NREGA), and the Food Security Act. One government committee after another declared that the levels of poverty in India were far higher than the Planning Commission would have us believe. India's health and human development indicators have dipped even below those of some sub-Saharan countries. Little wonder then that the virtues of primary health care are sought to be reinvented through the NRHM. These are however halting steps which do not demonstrate any desire on the part of the government to bring about a real paradigm shift. The National Health Mission (earlier NRHM plus Urban Health Mission) is in its second phase after extension beyond 2012. As already stated earlier, the goals and targets set for the first phase itself have remained elusive till date.

POST National Health Mission Scenario

The latest mantra in health care provisioning in the country is 'Universal Health Coverage' (UHC). Even though the formal policy remains undecided in this regard, but the deliberations regarding policy formulation for UHC provide valuable lessons in how vested interests and underlying ideological frameworks shape the development of the health services system.

We have already mentioned in the earlier chapter that the Planning Commission of India had set up a 'High Level Expert Group' (HLEG) to chalk out a path for achieving UHC in India. Surprisingly enough, contrary to the prevailing overall development thinking, the HLEG argued primarily for strengthening the public sector health services to provide UHC for the people. This however was not at the cost of oblivion of the private sector. The definition of UHC adopted by the expert group categorically stated – '....the government being the guarantor and enabler, although not necessarily the only provider of health-related services' (HLEG, 2011). Further, the recommendation 3.2.2 of the HLEG report categorically states—'Develop effective contracting in guidelines with adequate checks and balances for the provision of health care by the formal private sector' (Ibid.).

In our opinion placing reliance on strengthened public sector health services as the main recourse to accomplishing UHC is the most prudent, cost-effective and sustainable way to accomplishing UHC. However, there appears nothing in either the intent or the recommendations of HLEG to indicate an opposition to private providers partaking in its scheme. Yet, no sooner was the report out, the World Bank charged that the panel's recommendations advocated—'marginalization of the private sector' and the 'elimination of intermediation by insurance companies' (Dhar, 2011).

There are three issues related to such blatant interference by multilateral funding agencies like the World Bank—first, is national policy making the sovereign right of the Indian government; secondly, whose case is actually being argued through such interference; and last but not the least what are the consequences of this for the overwhelming majority of the working people of India?

As to the first issue, while the national policy making ought to be the sovereign right of India's government, but there are many instances to testify that the *oversized chests of Indian ruling politicians get deflated before their imperialist patrons.* Whose bidding the World

Bank was doing becomes clear from its observation—'There is a growing number of high-quality, low-cost providers that may be willing to engage with the government in providing defined packages of care to the poor. Policies need to be in place to foster more effective engagement with the private sector' (Dhar, 2011). HLEG's recommendation to eliminate intermediaries in the purchase of services from the private sector came in for special criticism from the Bank, especially as it thought that the insurance companies and other independent purchasing agencies had demonstrated substantial technical and organizational abilities in delivering these services (Dhar, 2011). As to what it means for the people, it shall be increasingly clarified through the chapters of this book.

That the Bank had successfully leveraged its position was amply reflected in the manner in which the government acted. An internal committee of the Planning Commission—the 'Steering Committee on Health for the Twelfth Five Year Plan (2012-2017)' that was constituted in May 2011 submitted its report in February 2012 (GOI, 2012), after the HLEG report in November 2011. If one were to believe the protestations of the health activists, the Steering Committee's recommendations effectively laid out a plan to hand over the country's health services system to the corporate sector (Dhar, 2012).

The mandarins at the Planning Commission already had their cue; at a meeting convened by the then prime minister's office on February 3, 2012, the Planning Commission berated the HLEG on charges that appeared imaginary and motivated. It was said:

> The (HLEG) report has not taken cognizance of the existence of a functioning health system built over decades, or assessed its potential or reasons for gaps, ... The HLEG report instead proposes creation of a new set-up for implementation of its goal... the HLEG has focused exclusively on UHC (universal health care) and, thereby, lacks holistic perspective (Makkar, 2012).

What is surprising is that the Steering Committee's observations and recommendations were what they were despite there being a fair sprinkling of academics and civil society representatives on its panel, which included luminaries like Binayak Sen, to include whom on the panel the Planning Commission ignored the protestations of the Chhattisgarh state government which had booked Sen under the draconian UAPA (unlawful activities prevention act) on charges of his being a sympathizer of the banned Communist Party of India (Maoist). Two of the members of the HLEG, including its Chairperson and convener were also members of the 'Steering Committee.' But it seems that the representatives of CII (Confederation of Indian Industries), FICCI (Federation of Indian Chambers of Commerce and Industry), ASSOCHAM (Associated Chamber of Commerce and Industry of India) and the Ccorporate Health Care carried far more weight than the rest. As Binayak Sen was to comment later at a symposium organized by the Centre for Social Medicine and Community Health at JNU that in the final meeting of the Steering Committee, while everyone else was given five minutes each to put across their point of view, Devi Shetty of Narayan Hrudayala, a leading light of corporate health care in the country, was privileged with a twenty-minute presentation. Whatever else may be the lessons here; these developments do convey a strong message regarding the potential of utilizing representation on the official forums for furthering the people's cause.

The whole affair only got murkier when in the face of opposition from various quarters to the proposals presented by the 'Steering Committee' it was decided by the Planning Commission to rework its report. However, it was only the language that was reworked, while the content remained the same. The result was what is now known as the 'July draft' that is said to have been prepared in consultation with the big shots of private health care industry—the head of Medanta Medicity in Gurgaon and chairperson of CII's national committee on health care, Naresh Trehan; the founder of Narayan Hrudayala, Devi Shetty; and the head of of Biocon Ltd in Bengaluru, Kiran Mazumdar Shaw (Pallavi et al., 2012).

Trehan has for long been an advocate of a clear division between 'provider and payer' where in the government should pay for purchasing health services from private providers. He reaffirmed – 'Government should stick to providing primary health care at state and district levels........ Specialty and super-specialty areas should be left to private sector since the government can afford neither the infrastructure nor the salaries to retain the talent required for tertiary care' (Makkar, 2012).

The problem is that the people only know it too well—how the interests of the poor are privileged by the for profit private sector, besides the fact that once the government's ability to provide services withers away, one need hardly hazard a guess to figure out who will be calling the shots.

Conclusion

From the Brettenwoods Conference to the economic meltdown of 2008, the world has indeed come a full circle. The question is however whether we wish to just keep moving round and round in circles. We have laid threadbare the anatomy of how the interests of the national and the international expropriating class have thwarted the aspirations of the labouring people of India to build a humane and just health system. The need is to defeat the conspiracy and break the circle.

The evolution of a health care system must be understood as a dialectical process that is impacted by almost every sphere of human activity. Therefore the solutions to the problems and challenges facing the development of a humane and just health care system can only be evolved through an understanding of this dialectics. This is frequently either not considered necessary by health professionals or is dealt with too casually as something that can be learned at any time. Rarely, if at all, do we see the functional utility of this understanding, and this is an attitude that must change.

Health is inherently a political issue. To address the problems facing it, what is essential is thorough going change in the underlying socio-economic and political conditions. One has to take sides; there is no middle path. Those of us, who stand for a health-care system free from the pervasive control of the market, need to align ourselves with the political forces working for systemic change. People'd health is too precious to be left to the tender mercies of the market. We can of course continue to remain bystanders, but only at the cost of our own dreams and health.

REFERENCES

Ablet, Jonathan, Adarsh Baijal, Eric Beinhocker et al. (2007): Executive Summary in 'The 'Bird of Gold', The Rise of India's Consumer Market.' McKinsey Global Institute, May.

Anstey, Vera (1945): 'Review: A Brief Memorandum Outlining a Plan of Economic Development for India', *International Affairs*, Vol. 21 (4): 556–7 .

Akanle, Oluwole (1992): Rescheduling of the External Debt: London Club, February 1992. United Nations Institute for Training and Research (UNITAR), February. Accessed on September 24, 2009 at http://www2.unitar.org/dfm/Resource_Center/Document_Series/Document1/C_Akanle.htm.

Burra, Arudra (2007): *The ICS and the Raj: 1919-50*, p. 3. Accessed at http://www.princeton.edu/~aburra/bv11feb07v1.2.pdf on September 23, 2009.

Backhouse, Roger E (2002): *The Penguin History of Economics* (Penguin), UK, pp. 236, 294-7.

Banerji, D. (2008): 'Concepts of Community Health', in '*Community Health Nursing*', Basavanthappa (ed.), 2 edn., (Jaypee Brothers), Delhi 2008, p. 43.

Burda, Michael and Charles Wyplosz (1997): *Macroeconomics: A European Text*, 2nd ed. (Oxford University Press), pp. 338–9.

Backhouse, Roger (2002): *The Penguin History of Economics* (Penguin), pp. 236, 294 – 7.

Boughton, James M (2001): 'Silent Revolution: The International Monetary Fund 1979–1989', International Monetary Fund. Accessed on September 25, 2009 at http://www.imf.org/external/pubs/ft/history/2001/index.htm.

BBC (1999): The NHS: the Conservative legacy, BBC News, September 20, Accessed on September 27, 2009 at http://news.bbc.co.uk/2/hi/health/background_briefings/your_nhs/85952.stm .

Bagchi, Amiya Kumar (Undated): 'Globalization: A Sketch', Centre for Peace and Development Studies. Accessed September 25, 2009 at http://www.cpdsindia.org/globalisationasketch.htm.

Chibber, Vivek (2003): '*Locked in Place: State-Building and Late Industrialization in India*', Princeton University Press, Princeton, p. 89.

Cueto, Marcos (2004): 'The Origins of Primary Health Care and Selective Primary Health Care', *Americal Journal Public Health*, November, 94(11): 1864–74.

Chaudhary, Praveen K., Vijay L. Kelkar, and Vikas Yadav (2004): 'The Evolution of "Homegrown Conditionality" in India: IMF Relations',

Journal of Development Studies, August, Vol. 40 (6): pp. 59–81.

Duggal, Ravi (2002): *Health Planning in India* (Rashtra Deepika Limited), *India Health: A Reference Document*, Kottayam, April, p. 6.

DeLong, J. Bradford (1998): Supply Shocks: The Dilemma of Stagflation', (University of California at Berkeley), accessed at http://econ161.berkeley.edu/multimedia/ASAD1.html. on September 23, 2009.

Daqing, Zhang and Paul U. Unschuld (2008): 'China's Barefoot Doctor: Past, Present, and Future', *Lancet* 372 (9653): 1865-7.

David Werner and Sanders David (1997): 'Chapter 3, Alma Ata and the Institutionalization of Primary Health Care, in, *Questioning the Solution: The Politics of Primary Health Care and Child Survival* (Health Wrights, Palo Alto, California), p. 19.

Duggal, Ravi (1998): Health Care and New Economic Policies: The Further Consolidation of the Private Sector in India, Paper Presented at the National Seminar on the Rights to Development, University of Mumbai, December 11-12, 1998) Mumbai: CEHAT, December Accessed on September 24, 2009 at http://www.cehat.org/publications/pa33a86.html.

Dhar, Aarti (2011): 'Panel on Health Coverage Addresses World Bank Concerns', *The Hindu*, 27 November.

Dhar, Aarti (2012): 'Activists Up in Arms Against New Proposal on Health care', *The Hindu*, August 8.

Gilmour, David (2007): '*The Ruling Caste: Imperial Lives in the Victorian Raj*', (Farrar, Straus, & Girard (Publishers)), New York.

Gindin, Sam (2002): 'Social Justice and Globalization: Are They Compatible?', *Monthly Review*, June, Vol. 54 (2).

Green, Duncan (2003): *Silent Revolution: The Rise and Crisis of Market Economics in Latin America* (New York University Press).

Government of India (2007): 'Report on Conditions of Work and Promotion of Livelihoods in the Unorganized Sector', National Commission for Enterprises in the Unorganized Sector accessed at http://nceus.gov.in/Condition_of_workers_sep_2007.pdf on September 24, 2009.

Government of India (2012): *'Report of the Steering Committee on Health for the Twelfth Five Year Plan'*, Health Division, Planning Commission, February.

Hansard (Record of the Proceeding of British Parliament) (1947 a): *India Transfer of Power*, H.C. Deb, June 3, 1947, Vol. 438 cc35-46, accessed at http://hansard.millbanksystems.com/commons/1947/jun/03/india-transfer-of-power#S5CV0438P0_19470603_HOC_251 on September 23, 2009.

Hansard, (1947 b): *Indian Independence Bill.* H.C. Deb, July 10, 1947, Vol. 439 cc2441-550, Accessed at http://hansard.millbanksystems.com/commons/1947/jul/10/indian-independence-bill#S5CV0439P0_19470710_HOC_289 on September 23, 2009.

Hazlitt, Henry (1959): 'The Failure of the New Economics', Ludwig von Mises Institute, accessed at http://mises.org/books/failureofnew economics.pdf on September 23, 2009.

Hall, Robert and John Taylor (1988): *Macroeconomics: Theory, Performance, and Policy* (2nd edition), (W.W. Norton & Co), New York.

Hughes, Gordon and Ross Furgusson (eds.) (2000): *Ordering Lives Family, Work and Welfare,* 2nd edn (Routledge & The Open University), London & New York, pp. 94-5.

Henales, Lidia and Beatrice Edwards (2002): 'Neoliberalism and Educational Reform in Latin America', *Current Issues in Comparative Education*, April 2002, Vol. 2(2), p. 2.

Hu, Vicky (2005): 'The Chinese Economic Reform and Chinese Entrepreneurship, in *X Jornada d'Economia de Caixa Manresa*. Accessed on September 26, 2009 at http://www.uoc.edu/symposia/caixamanresa/jornadaeconomia/2005/eng/vicky_hu.pdf .

HLEG (High Level Expert Group) (2011): 'High Level Expert Group Report on Universal Health Coverage for India', Planning Commission of India, November, p. 3.

Ibid., p. 16.

IMF Archives (undated): Finding Aids, Bretton Woods Conference Collection: Photographs. Accessed at http://www.imf.org/external/np/arc/eng/fa/BWC/s5.htm on September 24, 2009.

Johnson, Paul (1998): Margaret Thatcher, a champion of free minds and markets, she helped to dismantle the welfare state and make the world safer for capitalism. *The Times*, April 13. Accessed on September 23, 2009 at http://www.time.com/time/time100/leaders/profile/thatcher.html .

Kelkar, Vijay (2005): India's Economic Future: Moving Beyond State Capitalism, India Development Foundation, October. Accessed at www.gate4india.com/india.../download.html?...1186579903india%20economic%20future on September 23, 2009.

Kanagaratnam, K. (1979): 'A Review of the Bellagio Population and Health Papers', May 9, folder 'Health and Population', Rockefeller Foundation Archives, Rockefeller Centre, New York.

Krugman, Paul (2008): 'The Keynesian Moment', *New York Times*, November 29.

Lowenstein, Roger (2009). 'A Question of Numbers', *New York Times*, July 27, 2009. Accessed on September 26, 2009 at http://www.nytimes.

com/2005/01/16/magazine/16SOCIAL.html.

Macaulay, T. (1835): 'Macaulay's Minute on Indian Education, delivered on February 2, 1835 in the British Parliament. Accessed at http://www.columbia.edu/itc/mealac/pritchett/00generallinks/macaulay/txt_minute_education_1835.html on September 24, 2009.

Markwell, Donald (2006): *John Maynard Keynes and International Relations: Economic Paths to War and Peace* (Oxford University Press).

Makkar, Sahil (2012): 'Universal Health care Plan May Be Nixed', livemint.com; *The Wall Stree Journal*, February 23. Available from http://www.livemint.com/Articles/PrintArticle.aspx?eat=tp&artid=E54B1116-5BD7-11E1-BB2E-000B5DABF613 on February 25, 2012.

Prasad, C.S. (2007): *'Sixty Years of the Indian Economy 1947 to 2007' (Vol. 1)*, (New Century Publications), Delhi.

Perron, Pierre (1988): *The Great Crash, the Oil Price Shock and the Unit Root Hypothesis*, Princeton University and C.R.D.E, accessed from http://www.econ.princeton.edu/ERParchives/archivepdfs/M338.pdf. on 17 October 2009.

Pallavi, Aparna, Vibha Varshney, Alok Gupta (2012): *'Universal Health Scare', Down to Earth*, September 30. Available from http://www.downtoearth.org.in/coverage/universal-health-scare-39099 on December 17, 2015.

Ritu Priya (2005): 'Public Health Services in India: A Historical Perspective, in *Review of Health care In India,* ed. Leena V. Gangolli, Ravi Duggal, and Abhay Shukla, Centre for Enquiry into Health and Allied Themes, Research Centre of Anusandhan Trust, Survey No. 2804 & 2805, Mumbai.

Reagan, Ronald (1981): Presidential Inaugural Address, January 20, 1981. Accessed on September 26, 2009 at http://www.bartleby.com/124/pres61.html.

Singh, Manmohan (2005): 'Of Oxford, Economics, Empire, and Freedom', *The Hindu*, online edition dated July 10, 2005. Accessed at http://www.hindu.com/2005/07/10/stories/2005071002301000.htm on September 22, 2009.

Sullivan, Arhur and Steven M. Sheffrin (2003): *Economics: Principles in Action*, (Prentice Hall).

Thakurdas, Purushottam Das (1945): *A Brief Memorandum Outlining a Plan of Economic Development for India* (2 Vols.), (Penguin Books), London.

Thatcher, Margaret (1987): Interview for Woman's Own, September 23, 1987. Accessed on September 24, 2009 at http://www.margarett hatcher.org/speeches/displaydocument.asp?docid=106689.

UPI.com (1971): *Red China Admitted to UN*, accessed from http://www.upi.com/Audio/Year_in_Review/Events-of-1971/

12295509436546-1/#title on September 25, 2009.

Varman, Rohit and Ram Manohar Vikas (2007): 'Rising Markets and Failing Health: An Inquiry into Subaltern Health Care Consumption under Neoliberalism', *Journal of Macromarketing,* June, Vol. 27 (2): pp. 162-172.

Woodruff, Philip (1959): *The Men Who Ruled India: The Guardians,* (Jonathan Cape (Publishers)), London.

Wikipedia (undated): Vietnam War, accessed on September 24, 2009.

WHO and UNICEF (1978 a): Declaration of Alma-Ata. International Conference on Primary Health Care, Alma-Ata, USSR, September 6-12. Accessed on September 21, 2009 at http://www.who.int/hpr/NPH/docs/declaration_almaata.pdf.

WHO & UNICEF (1978 b): 'Primary Health Care: A Joint Report by The Director-General of the World Health Organization and The Executive Director the United Nations Children's Fund', Geneva, New York 1978, p. 11. Accessed on September 24, 2009 at http://whqlibdoc.who.int/publications/1978/9241541288_eng.pdf.

World Health Organization (WHO) (1981): Global Strategy for Health For All by the Year 2000, Geneva.

Walsh, J.A. and K.S. Warren (1979): 'Selective Primary Health Care: An Interim Strategy for Disease Control in Developing Countries', *New England Journal of Medicine, 1979;* 301: 967–74; it also appeared in *Social Science and Medicine,* 14C (1980): 145–63 as part of an issue devoted to the Bellagio meeting.

Wuyts, Marc (1998), 'Malthus, Then and Now: The Novelty of Old Ideas on Population and Economy', Dies Natalis address delivered on October 8, (Erasmus University Rotterdam), The Hague, Netherlands.

Zurbrigg, Sheila (1991): Chapter IV, 'Special Interests', in *Part III – 'Forces Shaping the Health System'* in *Rakku's Story: Structures of Ill-Health and the Source of Change* (Centre for Social Action), pp. 108-112.

Ibid., p. 107.

5

National Health Policy, 2017: Transition from a Draft Policy to Being the Official Prescription for Public Health Nemesis

This chapter has evolved in two phases. The Ministry of Health and Family Welfare put out the Draft National Health Policy (DNHP) in 2015 beginning for public debate. The initial part of this chapter i.e. the analysis of DNHP 2015 had been written as a response to the debate on DNHP on behalf of the faculty of Center for Social Medicine and Community Health, Jawaharlal Nehru University and was duly published in the *Economic and Political Weekly* (Rao et.al., 2015). This draft policy remained in a draft stage for more than two years. In the meanwhile the authors had proceeded with the process of publication of this book. Even as the book was almost ready to go to print, the National Health Policy 2017 was announced by the government. It was deemed necessary by the authors that the book should include a comment on the changes in the NHP 2017 over and above DNHP. This comment has been added here as a post script to the analysis of DNHP. Post script also seeks to assess the extent to which the debate on DNHP did or did not impact NHP 2017.

Both the public health analysis of DNHP 2015 and the comment on NHP 2017 by way of post script are being presented herewith sequentially for the readers.

THE 'DRAFT NATIONAL HEALTH POLICY, 2015' – A PUBLIC HEALTH ANALYSIS[1]

The Ministry of Health and Family Welfare, Government of India had put up its 'Draft Health Policy 2015' (DNHP) document for public debate, comments and suggestions. This critique is meant to contribute to this debate. In order to put the draft policy document in perspective, the first part deals with the economic, political and historical context of the present document; the second part highlights the basic premise and major recommendations of the draft policy; and the third critiques its major formulations.

Javid Choudhary and Anant Phadke (Choudhary, 2015; Phadke, 2015) have both contributed rich perspectives to the debate on DNHP. However, it is important here to mention the points of divergence and congruence between this critique and the opinions expressed by the two authors. Chaudhary introduces his submissions with the opinion:

> The National Health Policy 2015, which is in the process of being finalized, should, in place of the earlier "broadband" approach, adopt a "narrow focus" on primary health care through the National Rural Health Mission (NRHM). The latter has focused on primary health care and has shown visible results (Choudhary, 2015, p. 25).

This opinion essentially implies that DNHP ought to have taken the initiatives introduced as part of NRHM further by expanding their reach and making them more comprehensive. It may be noted that NRHM was designed for a specific purpose and as such cannot be a substitute for a 'National Health Policy' which by definition ought to cover entire gamut of issues impacting on health of the people and health care services. Not only did NRHM falter in achieving the goals set before it; but as is argued in this critique, its success has been marred by the larger trends that have come to

---

1. This comment on the Draft National Health Policy, 2015 had been published in the *Economic and Political Weekly* and full reference of this publication is - Mohan Rao, Prachin Godajkar, Rama Baru, Ramila Bisht, Ritu Priya Mehrotra, Rajib Dasgupta, Sunita Reddy, Vikas Bajpai (corresponding author). 'Draft National Health Policy 2015 - A Public Health Analysis', *Economic and Political Weekly*, April 25, 2015; Vol. 50 (17): 94 – 101.

dominate the health services system of the country. As such, the differentiation between *broadband approach* and *narrow focus* only on primary health care is artificial and could be counterproductive. Phadke, on the other hand, has concentrated on two important issues of 'strategic purchasing' of secondary and tertiary care services, an important recommendation of DNHP, and the regulation of the private health sector. Our critique discusses these issues, but brings forth very different aspects without entailing any repetition of views expressed by Phadke.

Economic, Political and Historical Context

This Draft Policy comes in the background of India having been witness to the implementation of the 'neoliberal' economic policies by different governments since 1990. Despite basic unity among the ruling classes on 'neoliberal economic policies', there have nevertheless been contestations among them over the issue of mitigating the adverse impact of these policies. These contestations were at play in the formulation of various social sector initiatives by the erstwhile UPA government. The announcement of National Rural Health Mission (NRHM) on the 12th of April 2005, with the intention of rejuvenating the rural health care in the country, was among the most important policy initiatives on the health front in recent history.

However, with the publication of the DNHP, health policy formulation in the country seems to have come to a full circle since the launching of NRHM. While the NRHM was preceded by extensive consultations, this has not been the case with the current document. As a consequence even the notional social-democratic considerations of the kind associated with formulation of NRHM were missing.

These are worrying signs and point towards an acceleration in consolidation behind the 'neoliberal development paradigm.' The disparate forms of this trend became increasingly concretized during the first decade of the new millennium. Beginning with the unanimous passage of the 'Special Economic Zone (SEZ)' Act in May 2005, the Indian Parliament has shown remarkable unity in passing major laws towards strengthening the legal framework for the implementation of neoliberal economic policies. The recent passage of 'Labour Laws - Exemption from Furnishing Returns and Maintaining Registers by Certain Establishments Amendment Bill, 2011' (*The Hindu*, 2014 a) and 'The Apprentices (Amendment) Bill, 2014' (*The Hindu*, 2014 b): in the Parliament by voice vote, without a single vote being cast against these, furnishes further proof of this unity.

The global economic crisis of 2008 was followed by the deceleration in the economic growth rates which contributed to the gloomy economic scenario both internationally and nationally. This has further added to the desperation in pursuit of elusive high economic growth by rendering ever more areas of the economy to maximization of profits by private capital. In this respect the potential of health care industry had been recognized early on. Recognizing this as an important context for the present draft policy, the document states:

> The second important change in context[2] is the emergence of a robust health care industry growing at 15% compound annual growth rate (CAGR). This represents twice the rate of growth in all services and thrice the national economic growth rate (MoHFW, 2014, p. 3).

It is further stated that:

> Indeed in one year alone 2012-13, as per market sources the private health care industry attracted over 2 billion dollars of FDI much of it as venture capital. For International Finance Corporation, the section of the World Bank investing in private sector, the Indian private health care industry is the second highest destination for its global investments in health (Ibid, p. 9).

These statements are potent tools of policy formulation designed to leverage the role of markets in health care that benefits the capital. Health and wellbeing of the people is thus incidental to this primary objective. The DNHP document thus privileges an economic agenda in health care rather than a public health agenda.

---

2. The draft policy document describes four important ways in which the context of health care has changed in the country viz. changes in the health priorities; emergence of robust health care industry; rise in catastrophic health expenditure due to health care costs; and increased fiscal capacity due to economic growth.

Overall Premise and Major Recommendations of the 'Draft National Health Policy 2015 '

Before going to the actual recommendations, it is important to understand the overall premise of the policy document. The draft policy document seems to proceed from two fundamental assumptions:

1. Firstly, barring some shortcomings, overall the policy initiatives taken subsequent to the 'National Health Policy 2002' have served us well, and that further development of the health services can be achieved by strengthening earlier initiatives and supplementing them with new policy initiatives.
2. Secondly, there seems to be an assumption of seamless continuity and harmony of purpose between the public and the private health care delivery systems which renders the latter amenable to achieve public health goals in health policy.

It is stated that among the various achievements made as a result of the previous policies have been a near total achievement of the MDGs (Millennium Development Goals) related to health; a substantial increase in the number of health personnel in the peripheral health services, especially an increase in the number of ASHAs (Accredited Social Health Activists) who have served as principal instrument for pushing the institutional delivery rates; and major increases in "outpatient attendance, bed occupancy and institutional delivery."

Another major achievement that is listed is in the area of 'publically financed health insurance schemes.' The document states:

> The population coverage under these various schemes increased from almost 55 million people in 2003-04 to about 370 million in 2014 (almost one-fourth of the population). Nearly two thirds (180 million) of this population are those in the Below Poverty Line (BPL) category. Evaluations show that schemes such as RSBY, have improved utilization of hospital services, especially in private sector and among the poorest 20% of households and SC/ST households (Ibid, 8).

The document is also forthcoming in acknowledging some of the shortcomings of the previous health policy initiatives. As regards NRHM it is stated:

> Much of the increase in service delivery was related to selective reproductive and child health services and to the national disease control programmes, and not to the wider range of health care services that were needed (Ibid, 6),
>
> While such a limited scope enabled progress in a few indicators, this was a poor strategy. Beyond a point, such selective facility development is neither sustainable nor efficient" (Ibid, 7).

Likewise, with respect to 'publically financed health insurance' it is stated:

> The insurance schemes vary widely in terms of benefit packages and have resulted in fragmentation of funds available for health care; especially selective allocation to secondary and tertiary care over primary care services. All National and State health insurance schemes need to be aligned into a single insurance scheme and a single fund pool reducing fragmentation (Ibid, 9).

These pronouncements however, ought to be seen in relation to the emphasis laid in the document – firstly over non-coverage of conditions like non-communicable diseases and injuries in the present set of interventions, and secondly, on the need to reduce the catastrophic out of pocket expenditures incurred both in public as well as private health facilities.

Hence, among its objectives the draft policy emphasizes the following (Ibid, 14 & 15):

- Significant reduction in out of pocket expenditures on health care to reduce incidence of catastrophic expenditures and consequent impoverishment.
- Apart from reproductive, maternal, child and adolescent health services, include care for most prevalent communicable and non-communicable diseases as free, comprehensive and universal primary health care entitlement.
- Universal access to free essential drugs, diagnostics, emergency ambulance services, and emergency medical and surgical care services.
- Improve the access to affordable secondary and tertiary

medical care through both public hospitals and their "strategic purchase" from private health sector.

- An "effective, efficient, rational, safe, affordable and ethical" health services system shall be sought to be developed by seeking to align the goals and objectives of private health care industry with public health goals.

The document seems to suggest that a health policy can broaden the ambit of services delivered through primary health care services while simultaneously reducing the catastrophic health expenditures through a policy of "strategic purchasing" of curative health services from both the public and private sectors, and that such a policy can enable India to achieve the goal of 'Universal Health Care.'

Major recommendations of Draft National Health Policy, 2015

The DNHP states its overall goal as:

> The attainment of highest possible level of good health and well-being, through a preventive and promotive health care orientation in all developmental policies, and universal access to good quality health care services without anyone having to face financial hardship as a consequence.

In order to achieve this, some of the major recommendations of the 'Draft NHP are:[3]

- **Primary care services and continuity of care (Ibid, 22 & 23):**
    - ➢ While the draft policy talks of 'up-grading existing health sub-centers' and orienting all primary health centers to provide *'comprehensive set of preventive, promotive, curative and rehabilitative services'* (emphasis ours), it simultaneously talks of delivering 'Comprehensive Primary Care' as an

---

3. We are mentioning here only those recommendations which in our opinion constitute the core thrust of the policy as distinct from the pre-existing public health interventions; or recommendations regarding aspects of health policy which are of structural importance to health services, irrespective of their novelty. Some other recommendations have been commented upon briefly in a separate subsection of the paper.

entitlement, wherein every family shall possess a health card that will link them to a primary care facility and be eligible for this *"package of services"* (emphasis ours)

- This *'package of services'* is to be delivered through suitably trained nurses and paramedical workers. For all chronic illnesses, it is proposed that once a treatment is started by a doctor/specialist at a higher facility, the continuance phase of treatment can be provided locally by the primary care team.
- The successful implementation of the package of *'primary care interventions'* shall be supported through a system of individual or team incentives and that ASHA shall have a crucial role in such implementation.
- The draft policy talks of referral linkages and support mechanisms for primary care facilities by leveraging their two way linkage with secondary and tertiary facilities through telemedicine and ICT.

- **Secondary and tertiary care services (Ibid, 24, 25 & 42):**
  - It is proposed to purchase the secondary and the tertiary care services both from the public sector as also the private sector facilities with public funds, either by the government directly or through national or state level intermediary institutional mechanisms like insurance agencies, trusts etc.
  - A concept of *'strategic purchasing'* has been introduced that refers to "the Government acting as a single payer-purchasing care from public hospitals and private providers as part of strategic plan for district health systems development." Another important aspect of *'strategic purchasing'* need be quoted here verbatim:

    "One element of strategic purchasing is that there is preference to public facilities – justified by the *needs of* national health programmes, many of which are not and never will be commercially remunerative; by the need to retain adequate reserve capacity for public health emergencies ....Even within private sector strategic preference for not for profit hospitals which are prepared to work on cost recovery principles and address public health goals in a spirit of service would require to be prioritized" (Ibid, 24).

- It is claimed that *'strategic purchasing'* shall help provide stewardship to private sector to develop itself for providing health services privileged by the state in strategic purchase.
- Vis-à-vis the public sector facilities it is proposed that while expenditure on core infrastructure facilities, human resources and supplies would be met through budgetary allocation; but an increasing part of resource allocation would be "responsive to quantity, diversity and quality of caseloads provided care."
- As a part of re-orienting public hospitals, it is proposed that rather than being viewed as providers of free health care, they shall be viewed as part of a 'tax financed single payer health care system' where in they shall be remunerated through pre-payment akin to commercial insurance – a method that has been deemed as *'cost effective'* in provisioning of population's health care needs.

- **Infrastructure Development**
  - With regard to infrastructure development the policy makes a very important shift – "From normative approaches in their development to targeted approaches to reach under-serviced areas," (p. 20) wherein "a conscious effort shall be made to identify districts and blocks which have the larger gaps for development of infrastructure and deployment of additional human resources" (p. 25).
  - The policy also seeks to achieve a measurable improvement in the quality of care in public health facilities with certification from competent boards. It is also intended to incentivize the facilities showing a measurable improvement in this regard (p. 26).

- **Human resources for health (pp. 37 & 38)**

  Some of the important recommendations in this regard are:
  - The government intends to strengthen the existing 58 medical colleges and upgrade district hospitals in further 58 districts to medical colleges.

- To fulfill the requirement of faculty for these medical colleges and provide personnel for high quality biomedical research, it is proposed that the number of AIIMS like institutions shall be increased from 9 to 15.
- It is proposed that the "rules regarding setting up of medical colleges and the entire system of regulation of medical education would also be informed and guided by the needs of correcting the current distortions of medical educational policy that have led to this mismatch between needs and skills."
- Apart from measures like attractive pay scales, better living and service conditions etc. it is proposed to give preference to students from underserved areas, in the hope that they shall be willing to go back to serve in these areas. More rural location of medical colleges, modification in curriculum and pedagogy of medical education are some other measures being thought of to motivate doctors to work in disadvantaged communities.
- A slew of measures have been proposed to enhance the training of specialists and to increase the availability of personnel from paramedical disciplines and AYUSH for taking care of curative needs of the people in primary care settings, by introducing various bridge courses to impart them necessary skills.

How likely are these policy prescriptions to succeed?

Health is produced in the social, economic, political and cultural context of a given society. It is only natural then that the recommendations of the draft policy should be analyzed within the prevailing social, economic and political context of the country.

There are two principle contradictions that bedevil the development of health services in the country and the public health outcomes resulting there from. These are:

1. Contradiction between the private sector health care, with corporatized tertiary care hospitals as its highest form, and the public sector health care (including all primary, secondary and tertiary care institutions) to leverage the health care needs of the people.

2. Contradiction between the health care needs of the affluent sections and the health care needs of the masses i.e. class interests in health care provisioning.

These contradictions are formative for other contradictions in the delivery of health care services, such as between preventive and curative care; between rural and urban; between primary and secondary/tertiary levels of care; between pre/para-clinical disciplines and clinical disciplines and those between different clinical disciplines themselves.

The policy planners have tried to resolve these principle contradictions by negating their very existence. Their argument is:

- Both public and private sector can be leveraged towards fulfilling the public health needs of India (Ibid; MoHFW, 2002).
- There is no contradiction between providing for the health care needs of the affluent and the poor; and that the government is fully committed towards providing affordable health care for the poor.

However these arguments deserve a closer scrutiny.

Relationship between the public and private sectors

To borrow from Chinese leader Deng Xiaoping's famous maxim - "It doesn't matter whether a cat is white or black, as long as it catches mice;" one might argue—'how does it matter whether it is public or private sector health care so long as it successfully caters to the health needs of the people?' Meanwhile, we need remember that Deng Xiaoping led the establishment of 'Market Socialism' in China.

The supposed harmony between the public and private sectors, of which Public-Private Partnerships (PPPs) are a specific form, is the new age panacea constructed at the end of 1990s. These partnerships were initiated to circumvent the problems created by blanket privatization of the development sector under neoliberal economic policies. The IMF in its policy paper of March 2004 on PPPs stated the following:

> By the late 1990s privatization was losing much of its earlier momentum, yet concerns about infrastructure remained in many

> countries. It was at this time that PPPs began to emerge significantly as a means of obtaining private sector capital and management expertise for infrastructure investment, both to carry on where privatization had left off and as an alternative where there had been obstacles to privatization. (IMF, 2004, p. 4).

There is an irreconcilable conflict between the very motives of the 'private' and 'public' sectors – the motive of *'profit maximization'* of the private sector, and the *'need to serve all irrespective of the ability to pay'* of the public sector, which precludes any symbiotic relationship between the two. Public health sector is entirely dependent on public resources and government patronage for its nourishment. But when the government itself is committed to see the expansion of the private sector, the relationship between the two sectors becomes outright parasitic wherein the private sector flourishes at the cost of enfeebling the public sector. The formal pronouncements of commitment towards strengthening public sector are meant only for public consumption.

In terms of government encouragement and committing public resources towards the growth of private health sector, the health policy draft states that:

> The Government has had an active policy in the last 25 years of building a positive economic climate for the health care industry. Amongst these measures are lower direct taxes; higher depreciation in medical equipment; Income tax exemptions for 5 years for rural hospitals; custom duty exemptions for imported equipment that are lifesaving; Income tax exemption for Health Insurance; and active engagement through publicly financed health insurance which now covers almost 27% of the population. Further forms of assistance are preferential and subsidized allocation of land that has been acquired under the public acquisition Act, and the subsidized education for medical, nursing and other paramedical professional graduating from government institutions and who constitute a significant proportion of the human resources that work for the private sector;.... (MoHFW, 2014, p. 9).

Contrary to this, under the sub-heading 2.8—'NRHM as an instrument for strengthening state health systems', the state of affairs has been acknowledged as follows:

> The National Rural Health Mission was intended to strengthen State health systems to cover all health needs, not just those of the national

> health programme. In practice, however it remained confined largely to national programme priorities...... Strengthening health systems for providing comprehensive care required higher levels of investment and human resources than were made available. The budget received and the expenditure there under was only about 40% of what was envisaged for a full re-vitalization in the NRHM Framework (p. 7).

There have been instances when even the programmatic interventions under NRHM, became an excuse for privileging the private health sector, rather than strengthening the public sector rural health care. In the year 1992 the State of Uttar Pradesh launched a public-private partnership named Merrygold scheme, based on a 'Social Franchising Model' (UP NRHM, 2013). In its PIP (Programme Implementation Plan) for the year 2013-14 submitted to the Ministry of Health and Family Welfare, Government of India, one of the objectives of Merrygold scheme was:

> To provide choice of services of assured quality to people at affordable pre fixed prices and thereby *shifting the workload of public health facilities* (UP NRHM, 2013).

The role of NRHM in the scheme was described as:

- Accreditation of the franchised hospitals with the Government health schemes i.e. JSY scheme and Family Planning.
- Linkage of ASHA Workers with each franchised facility for client referrals (UP NRHM, 2013).

So the services that were to be provided by a strengthened public health apparatus was, ended up being opened to the private sector, subsidized by public money, in the name of providing a *'choice of services'* (emphasis ours); and ASHA, the *'social health activist'* was turned into the agent for bolstering private health care industry.

In the year 2013, the State of Uttarakhand outsourced 16 of its best CHCs to private for profit sector for fully operationalizing their services. What is noteworthy is that as per the terms of reference of the contract, the state government assured 15 per cent profit for the operators irrespective of the number of footfalls at the facilities. Further, the operator was to provide only the clinical services and had no responsibility for implementing preventive and promotive functions or the national health programs (Bajpai, 2014).

The phenomenon of non compliance by many corporate hospitals, of their obligation to treat poor patients free of charge despite availing of huge public subsidies has been well documented (Qureshi Committee). However, in a remarkable example of how the government is willing to privilege the 'profit' interest over the public interest, the draft policy document states:

> Given that the private sector operates within the logic of the market and that they contribute to the economy through their contribution to the growth rate and by the national earnings from medical tourism, there need not be any major effort to persuade them to care for the poor, as long as their requirements and perceptions do not influence public policy towards universal health care (p. 36).

But, have their *'requirements and perceptions'* not already influenced public policy in so far as such a statement finds place in the 'National Health Policy' document?

Corporate hospitals today they have come to occupy the 'commanding heights'[4] of medical practice in the country; a place that not so long ago was reserved for medical college hospitals. As a consequence of this the motto of earning super profits from human misery due to disease, in place of earning a decent living by rendering the necessary services, has come to be recognized as a legitimate goal of medical practice. This dislodged medical profession from its ethical roots in serving the society. The overall objective of maximizing profits and absolute answerability to share holders imposes a political economy of medical practice that has the following consequences.

Curative care must be privileged over preventive and promotive care leading to the neglect of the social determinants of health.

Within curative care, high end technologies, irrespective of their desirability and affordability must be privileged even if simpler, effective, efficient and affordable technologies are available. Such pattern of care privileges the health care needs of the rich over those of the poor.

4. While the heights attained by these hospitals in terms of rational treatment and medical ethics are circumspect, they have certainly defined the heights of technology driven treatments irrespective of their desirability and the glamour associated with corporate medical practice.

This pattern of care also places its demands on the content of medical education; it moulds the career choices and ethical moorings of medical graduates. Today the skill sets of the graduates and post-graduates passing from our medical colleges makes them feel more at home in the better equipped medical facilities of the cities, or indeed the "world class" hospitals in U.S. or U.K., rather than in a rural PHC (Primary Health Centre) or CHC (Community Health Centre) in India.

Privileging curative care also fuels the pursuit of specialization and super-specialization in clinical disciplines at the cost of preventive and socialized medicine. A health services system geared to cater to the needs of the affluent in the main, seeks to enhance the monopoly of the elite over the medical profession such that there is little dichotomy between the aspirations of medical professionals and the overall objectives of the market oriented health services system they serve. The rapid spurt in private medical colleges is but a consolidation of this trend. The few recruits from marginalized regions or communities who may find entry into the profession may find their love for their region or their community too weak to stand up to the dominant moorings of the system, for compliance with the latter is essential for their rise in the system (Ananthakrishnan, 2010).

Domination of the market in the health care system of the country is both systemic and systematic. The multi-specialty hospitals of the bigger cities are linked up with smaller nursing homes, doctors and employees in the public health facilities, private clinics, formal and non-formal medical practitioners down to the level of mofussil towns and districts to ensure a steady supply of patients. There is a well oiled system of cuts and commissions and agents. (Nagral, 2014; Nundy, 2014; Gadre, 2015).

A viable public sector is a threat to the hegemony of the private sector; hence, it is imperative that public health services be undermined. Starving public facilities of funds, stopping recruitment altogether or recruiting personnel on contractual basis and unattractive wages such that the best talent is kept out, poor supply of material are just some of the measures adopted to set in demoralization among the public sector health workers and reduce the functionality of services. Public health facilities have also been undermined by engraining commercial principles and processes in their functioning through commercialization of their services.

This however does not mean that no form of private sector can be harnessed for achieving public health goals. The NHS (National Health Service) of United Kingdom, where the system utilizes the services of many general practitioners integrated with the national health system, in order to meet the primary level health care needs of the people. But, a highly regulated private practice and the public health services continuing to define the 'commanding heights' of medical practice is a necessary condition to achieve such collaboration between the public and the private sector.

Lessons of the practices since NHP 2002

As pointed above, one of the assumptions underlying the premises of this policy has been that of post NHP 2002 policy interventions having been largely successful. Of the successes that have been prominently mentioned in the draft policy document are achieving MDGs with respect to maternal and child mortality along with related rise in rates of institutional deliveries; and a wide expansion of publically provided health insurance which seems to have hugely powered the most prominent recommendation of the present policy – 'strategic purchasing' of secondary and tertiary level health services.

MDGs and the Package of RCH Related Interventions

From the evidence that is available, attribution of decline in MMR and child mortality to the package of interventions in RCH (reproductive and child health) is highly circumspect. Firstly, there is no evidence to show a direct correspondence between the two at All India level. Rather, in the case of the state of Uttar Pradesh a steep rise in the rates of institutional deliveries has been accompanied with slower decline in the rates of infant and maternal mortality; with this slowdown being particularly sharp for the latter (Bajpai, undated).

The network of sub-centers, PHCs, CHCs and district hospitals in the country meant to cater to the health care needs of rural India might be huge, but there are serious questions regarding the level of functionality of these facilities and the quality of services rendered by them even with regard to the limited services offered by them.

Table 1 below gives us an idea of functional status and quality of care available in rural health care facilities. All CHCs, as conceived to begin with, were to provide secondary level care with specialist consultation in all basic clinical disciplines and were to function as the First Referral Point (FRU) for various kinds of emergencies. However, the non-availability of specialists in many of these disciplines has compromised their ability to perform these functions. At All India level only about 52 per cent of the CHCs were designated as FRUs and only 18.7% were providing Caesarean section facility even though 25 per cent of the CHCs were having the services of an obstetrician; and of the CHCs providing Cesarean section services, less than half had blood storage facility, without which to perform C section is fraught with immense risk. One can likewise read the data of some of the other north Indian EAG (Empowered Action Group) states to draw appropriate conclusions. Such discrepancies can lead to situations where the services cannot be delivered despite physical infrastructure being there, either because the doctor, or some other facility like the blood storage facility is not there; else non-dependability of electricity supply due to missing power back-up renders them dysfunctional. As a result, the system operates sub-optimally.

Table 1: Infrastructure, Staff and Services at CHC (%)

India/State	*Obs. & Gyne.*	*24 hr normal delivery services*	*Funct-ional operation theatre*	*Desig-nated as FRUs*	*Designated as FRUs offering cesa-rean section*	*New born care on 24 hour basis*	*Blood storage facility*
India	25.2	90.0	65.2	52	18.7	76.1	9.1
Bihar	40.9	90.9	86.4	87.9	18.8	72.4	0.0
Chhattisgarh	19.7	99.3	73.0	56.9	22.1	80.8	7.7
Jharkhand	62.5	100.0	87.5	87.5	0.0	85.7	0.0
Madhya Pradesh	15.8	99.6	70.7	61.4	17.7	86.2	6.3
Odisha	87.3	79.0	59.4	53.7	15.5	53.7	15.5
Rajasthan	29.9	98.9	60.3	52.7	38.0	88.2	15.0
Uttar Pradesh	19.5	92.1	88.5	55.8	6.2	71.8	1.3

Source: Government of India (2013)

A number of civil society groups got together to bring out a report – 'Dead Women Talking' on 124 maternal deaths reported from 10 different states. Of the total number of maternal deaths, 60 per cent had managed to reach a medical facility in face of complication, whereas 60 women died in medical facilities, of which 48 died in public health facilities while 12 died in private facilities; 22 women died while travelling from one facility to another. There were heart rending stories of public health institutions referring women in distress to higher facilities without even having a look at the dying woman (Subha Sri B and Khanna R, 2014). The recent death of 13 women, all in their 20s and 30s, in a family planning sterilization camp organized at Bilaspur, is another case in point (SAMA, JSA & NAMHHR, 2014).

These stark findings notwithstanding, with respect to health infrastructure and manpower development DNHP talks of moving *"from normative approaches in their development to targeted approaches to reach under-serviced areas."* Taken in the totality of things, this is nothing but an admission of the fact that "since we cannot meet the norms, we shall emphasize reaching under-serviced areas in a targeted manner. Rationale for targeting could have existed if the need was to address underdeveloped public health services only in some geographical pockets, in an overall reasonably well performing public health system; this however is not the case with respect to India where the malady is far more pervasive.

Experience of Publically Funded Health Insurance with Private Service Provisioning

It would be prudent to point here some of the important pitfalls of publically financed health insurance schemes as a caution against overoptimistic reliance on them to achieve the goals of draft national health policy. Providing protection against catastrophic out of pocket expenditure has been the stated rationale of implementing publically financed health insurance schemes; however, available evidence shows that undermining financial protection for the poor is precisely what these schemes end up doing.

A study by Selvaraj and Karan regarding impact of Rashtriya Swasthya Beema Yojana (RSBY), Rajiv Aarogyasri (RAS) in Andhra Pradesh (A.P.), and Tamil Nadu Health Insurance schemes on out of pocket expenditure showed that poorer households in the districts where these schemes were implemented ended up having higher out of pocket expenditure, including catastrophic expenditure, as compared to poor households in districts where these schemes were not implemented (Selvaraj S and Karan A K, 2012). In Andhra Pradesh the annual budget spent under the Rajiv Arogyasri scheme on surgeries in private hospitals was higher than that spent in tertiary care public hospitals, but that the private hospital associations, by threatening to withdraw from the scheme bargained for higher costs to be paid to them. Hence, while the profits were privatized; the losses were socialized, besides rendering such schemes untenable in the long run (Reddy and Mary, 2013; Prasad and Raghavendra, 2012). The list of problems thrown up in the implementation of these schemes – moral hazards, unnecessary diagnostic tests, the spate of hysterectomies etc. is indeed too long to be summarized here.

Pointing to the huge cost to public health on account of RAS scheme in A.P., the former health secretary to the Government of India wrote:

> Among 19 major States, Andhra Pradesh incurred the lowest expenditure of Central grants (National Rural Health Mission and disease control programmes) as proportional to its total health spending during 2011; 16 per cent against 31 and 28 percentages by Maharashtra and Karnataka respectively and the only State to slash its primary care budgets from 53 per cent to 46 per cent and allocate just 9 per cent for secondary care down from 12 per cent during 2007-12. In comparison, RAS was provided 23 per cent of the health budget for less than 1 per cent of the population (not necessarily poor) or 11.3 per cent of total hospitalization (Rao, 2014).

These health insurance schemes are only payment mechanisms which fail to account for a number of non-financial barriers that temper the impact of these schemes on out of pocket expenditure, such as – regional and rural-urban imbalance in the socioeconomic development and the consequent imbalance in the development of health services, the connectivity of a place to health facilities and the availability of efficient means of transport, the literacy status of the people, their confidence and trust in the available health facilities (Narasimhan et. al, 2014; Bajpai and Saraya, 2012).

What remains unacknowledged by the policy planners is that these schemes are nothing but a sort of reverse cash transfer of public money for ensuring mega profits for the corporate driven health care (Rao, 2014; Prasad and Raghvendra, 2012; *The Hindu*, 2007).

A Word About Some of the Recommendations of the Draft Policy

- ***Comprehensive versus package of services:***

On one hand the policy promises to deliver a *'comprehensive set of preventive, promotive, curative and rehabilitative services'* through the sub-centers and the PHCs, and at the same time talks of a *"package of services"* – the contradiction between the terms 'comprehensive' and 'package of services' is self evident.

Moreover, this 'package' is to be delivered by suitably trained nurses and paramedical workers, implying that the role of trained physicians stands to be further marginalized at primary level of care, which means that the part care that is not within the 'package' e.g. components of curative care shall be even more difficult to provide at primary level. This can act as a barrier to enhancing the credibility of public health institutions in the eyes of common people and hence a reason for continued reliance on the private sector.

- ***Commercial financing mechanism for public hospitals:***

Other than the regular budgetary support for manpower and infrastructure, it is proposed to provide budgetary support for the services of a public hospital through the mechanism of a 'commercial insurance scheme.' This is meant to bring the operations of public hospitals on same commercial footing as those of the private hospitals contracted in by the government through 'strategic purchasing.' Given the trend of privileging of private health care in publically financed health insurance schemes; this sets the stage for quietly shifting greater part of the budgetary support to private sector at a later date.

Under RSBY there were 3,200 private and 1,100 public hospitals were enrolled throughout India (Basu, Undated). Likewise the bulk of business under the Rajiv Arogyasri Scheme went to the private sector (Shukla et. al, 2011).

- ***Abolition of user charges and provision of free medicines in public hospitals***

This by far is the most welcome of the proposals in the draft policy document. However, the extent to which this will be able to provide relief to the people will depend on whether drugs shall be free and user charges will be exempt only for the predefined 'package of services' or for all conditions. If there is large scale outsourcing of services to private sector, this might only end up increasing the out of pocket expenditure besides further deterioration in the services rendered by public sector.

It need be remembered that, even though there has been reduction in out of pocket expenditure on institutional deliveries due to implementation of Janani Sishu Suraksha Karyakram (JSSK); the institutional delivery program has not managed to entirely wipe it out (Govil et. al, undated; Tripathi et. al, 2014; Modugu et. al, 2012) Even the conditional success of JSSK could be possible because it were the public health services that shouldered the major responsibility for this and not the private sector.

- ***Social determinants of health:***

DNHP appropriately lays emphasis on "holistic approach and cross sectoral convergence in addressing social determinants of health" including 'measurable achievements' to be achieved through planned and adequately financed institutional mechanisms" (MoHFW, 2014, pp. 17-18) to improve the 'environment for health.' However, apart from placing reliance on 'Swachh Bharat Abhiyan' and the ICDS (Integrated Child Development Scheme), there is absence of other initiatives in this regard.

Intersectoral coordination has largely remained a non starter in health sector. It would have helped if the policy reflected on the past experience in this regard to prime the health sector taking initiative in bringing about such a coordinated functioning. Instead DNHP reduces health sector to the role of only undertaking "evidence based advocacy within Government and in the media" (Ibid, 17) to highlight the link between social determinants and disease. Recognizing the centrality of social determinants of health, authors have even called for a specific sub-cadre for facilitating action in this regard (Ritu Priya and Chikersal, 2013).

- ***AYUSH:***

The principal problem regarding the alternative/Indian systems of medicine is their being regarded as a poor substitute to allopathic medicine. It has taken a long time since the 1946 Health Survey and Development Committee Report (Bhore Committee Report) for ending the official apartheid against the indigenous systems at least at the level of policy; however, this apartheid seems to continue in practice despite repeated assurances of strengthening educational, curative and research institutions in this stream. The policy fails to suggest measures to break this log jam, even though it reposes faith in the potential for AYUSH to strengthen the preventive and promotive aspects of health apart from its curative potential.

However, it is to the document's credit that it gives more space and emphasis on folk medicine beyond the textual systems, and that is a welcome shift that recognizes people's knowledge as a people empowering measure.

- ***Institutional mechanisms:***

Even on a preliminary reflection it is difficult to lose sight of the fact that the countries where insurance driven model of health care provisioning works with any measure of efficiency, have a highly regulated health sector, while in India private health sector is almost unregualted. In fact the very character of private health sector poses immense difficulties in its regulation (Baru, 2013). In countries like U.S.A., despite regulation, much is left to be desired in terms of fulfilling public health objectives.

We would not further elaborate on this issue as the same has already been discussed in Phadke's article (Phadke, 2015).

Concluding Remarks

National Health Policy 2015 Draft document actually amounts to dismembering the complex process of health policy formulation in a hugely diverse country like India. Over riding this diversity, it adopts a 'one solution suits all' approach by decisively pushing insurance based health care model for facilitating a near monopoly of the corporate sector in curative care. Much is being made of the possibilities of harnessing private health care for achieving public health goals; however, the fundamental contradiction between the objectives of private and public health sectors, which is too powerful to be undone by theoretical formulations.

A huge body of evidence that negates the feasibility of DNHP recommendations has been conveniently ignored. Given the political and economic environment obtaining in the country today, this is not an inadvertent omission. Complex national and international forces have been at work in shaping the present idea of 'Universal Health Care' which is a cruel distortion of the first attempt made by the international community to achieve 'Universal Health Care' for the people of the world through a much more holistic approach of 'Primary Health Care' (Bisht, 2013). Rather than alleviate the suffering of the poor man and woman due to disease, this policy has every potential to become the quintessential mill stone around their necks. As Qadeer has put it:

A model of Universal Health Care based on public private partnerships [PPPs] in the form public financing and private delivery, focusing on universal access to an essential health package while keeping silent on tertiary care, will ultimately strengthen the for profit health sector at the cost of the public health care services and undermine access to care for the marginalized (Qadeer, 2013).

The final results would depend on the rigor with which pro-people health professionals, academics, activists and people oppose the pro-business formulations of DNHP.

REFERENCES

Ananthakrishnan N (2010): 'Medical education in India: Is it still possible to reverse the downhill trend?' *National Medical Journal of India*, Vol. 23 (3): 156-160.

Bajpai V (undated): Manuscript No. IJSW/BX-1/13/63 - 'Implementation of Janani Sishu Suraksha Karyakram (JSSK) in Uttar Pradesh – Some Observations and Concerns', *Indian Journal of Social Work* on January 19, 2015.

Bajpai V (2014): 'Reluctance of medical personnel to work in rural areas and the imperative to functionalize peripheral health services; are public private partnerships the answer: an evaluation of the proposal to give community health centers (CHCs) on ppp mode in Uttrakhand

State of India. *Global Journal of Public Health and Medicine*, Vol. 3 (2).

Bajpai V and Saraya A (2012): 'Rashtriya Swasthya Beema Yojna: A Public Health Perspective,' *Indian Journal of Social Work*, Vol. 73 (2): 265–286.

Basu R (Undated): 'Rashtriya Swasthya Bima Yojana: Pioneering Public-Private Partnership in Health Insurance,' Network of Asia-Pacific Schools and Institutes of Public Administration and Governance. Available from http://www.napsipag.org/PDF/RUMKI%20 BASU.pdf on February 1, 2015.

Baru R (2013): 'Challenges for Regulating the Private Health Services in India', *Indian Journal of Public Health*, Vol. 57 (4): 208-211.

Bisht R (2013): 'Universal Health Care: The Changing International Discourse', *Indian Journal of Public Health*, Vol. 57 (4): 236-241.

Choudhary Javid (2015): 'National Health Policy 2015; A Narrow Focus Needed', *Economic and Political Weekly*, Vol. 50 (9): 25-30.

Government of India (2013): 'Table G – 2, Infrastructure, staff and services at CHC (%)' in *Health and Family Welfare Statistics India 2013*, Ministry of Health and Family Welfare, New Delhi.

Govil D, Purohit, Neetu, Gupta, S.D. (Undated): 'An Asesment of Out of Pocket Expenditure on Child Bearing Proces Post Janani Suraksha Yojana: A Case from Rajasthan, India,' International Union for Scientific Study of Population. Available from: http://iussp.org/sites/default/files/event_call_for_papers/Dipti%20Govil%20-%200967(1).pdf on February 1, 2015.

Gadre A (2015): 'India's private health care sector treats patients as revenue generators', *BMJ*; 350: h826.

International Monetary Fund (2004): 'Public-Private Partnerships,' prepared by Fiscal Affairs Department (In consultation with other departments, the World Bank, and the Inter-American Development Bank), March 12. Available from http://www.imf.org/external/np/fad/2004/pifp/eng/031204.pdf on 29th January 2014.

Ministry of Health and Family Welfare (MoHFW) (2014): 'National Health Policy 2015, Draft', New Delhi, December, p. 3.

Ibid., p. 9.

Ibid., p. 8.

Ibid., p. 6.

Ibid., p. 7.

Ibid., p. 9.

Ibid., pp. 14 & 15.

Ibid., pp. 22 & 23.

Ibid., pp. 24, 25 & 42.

Ibid., p. 20.

Ibid., p. 25.

Ibid., p. 26.

Ibid., pp. 37 & 38.

Ministry of Health and Family Welfare (2002): 'National Health Policy 2002', New Delhi.

Ministry of Health and Family Welfare (MoHFW) (2014): 'National Health Policy 2015, Draft', New Delhi, December, p. 9.

Ministry of Health and Family Welfare (MoHFW) (2014): 'National Health Policy 2015, Draft', New Delhi, December, p. 36.

Modugu H R, Kumar M, Kumar A, Millett C. (2012): 'State and socio-demographic group variation in out-of-pocket expenditure, borrowings and Janani Suraksha Yojana (JSY) programme use for birth deliveries in India.' *BMC Public Health*. 2012 Dec 5;12:1048. doi: 10.1186/1471-2458-12-1048.

Ministry of Health and Family Welfare (MoHFW) (2014): 'National Health Policy 2015, Draft', New Delhi, December, pp. 17, 18.

Ibid., 17.

Ibid., 44.

Ibid., 42.

Nagral S (2014): 'Corruption in Indian Medicine or 'Overenthusiasm of the Marketing Department.' *Economic and Political Weekly*, Vol. 49 (29).

Nundy S (2014): 'Corruption in Indian Medicine', *Current Medicine Research and Practice*, Vol. 4, Issue 3, Pages 99–100.

Narasimhan H, Boddu, V., Singh, P. et. al. (2014): 'Access to the Rajiv Aarogyasri community health insurance scheme of Andhra Pradesh,' *Health, Culture and Society*, Vol. 6 (1), DOI 10.5195/hcs.2013.163.

Phadke A (2015): 'Slippery Slope for Public Health Services', *Economic and Political Weekly*, Vol. 50 (9): 30-32.

Prasad N P and P. Raghvendra (2012): 'Health care Models in the Era of Medical Neo-liberalism: A Study of Aarogyasri in Andhra Pradesh,' *Economic and Political Weekly*, Vol. 47 (43): 118 – 126.

Qadeer I (2013): 'Universal health care in India: Panacea for whom?' *Indian Journal of Public Health*, Vol. 57 (4): 225-30.

Reddy S and Mary I (2013): 'Rajiv Aarogyasri Community Health Insurance Scheme in Andhra Pradesh, India: A Comprehensive Analytic View of Private Public Partnership Model', *Indian Journal of Public Health*, Vol. 57 (4): 254-259.

Rao S (2014): 'For public health as political priority', *The Hindu*, October 13.

Ritu Priya and Chikersal A (2013): 'Developing a public health cadre in 21 st century India: Addressing gaps in technical, administrative and social dimensions of public health services', *Indian Journal of Public Health*, Vol. 57 (4): 219-224.

Subha Sri B and Khanna R (2014): 'Dead Women Talking: A civil society report on maternal deaths in India,' Common Health and Jan Swasthya Abhiyan.

SAMA, JSA and NAMHHR (2014): 'Camp of Wrongs: The Mourning Afterwards, A fact finding report on sterilization deaths in Bilaspur,' November 27.

Selvaraj S and Karan A K (2012): 'Why Publicly-Financed Health Insurance Schemes Are Ineffective in Providing Financial Risk Protection', *Economic and Political Weekly*, Vol. 47 (11): 60 – 68.

Shukla R, Veena Shatrugna, R Srivatsan (2011): 'Aarogyasri Health care Model: Advantage Private Sector,' *Economic and Political Weekly*, Vol. 46 (49): 38-42.

The Hindu (2014 a): 'RS passes Bill amending labour Laws', November 26. Available from: http://www.thehindu.com/news/national/rs-passes-bill-amending-labour-laws/article6634231.ece on 26th Nov 2014.

The Hindu (2014 b): 'Parliament passes Apprentices Bill', November 27. Available from: http://www.thehindu.com/news/national/parliament-passes-apprentices-bill/article6637197.ece on 27th Nov 2014.

The Hindu (2007): 'Rajiv Arogya Sri scheme benefits corporates', August 20. Available from http://www.thehindu.com/todays-paper/tp-national/tp-andhrapradesh/rajiv-arogya-sri-scheme-benefits-corporates/article1895474.ece on January 31, 2015.

Tripathi N, Sushma Kumari Saini and Shankar Prinja (2014); 'Impact of Janani Shishu Suraksha Karyakram on Out-of-pocket Expenditure among Urban Slum Dwellers in Northern India,' *Indian Pediatrics*, 51: 475-477.

UP NRHM (2013): 'Annexure Merrygold, state level' made available by the state along with Uttar Pradesh State Program Implementation Plan for the year 2013-14 submitted to the Ministry of Health and Family Welfare, Government of India.

POSTSCRIPT TO DRAFT NATIONAL HEALTH POLICY 2015

This postscript is necessitated by the government's decision to finally come out with the health policy document titled 'National Health Policy 2017' (NHP 2017) after a long hiatus (MOHFW, 2017 a). Since it took unusually long for the policy document to be finalized it was expected that it would embody some of the suggestions originating from the rich discussion around the draft policy document. However, it is disappointing that the concerns which had been raised in our earlier critique remain unaddressed in the final policy. It can hardly be a matter of any satisfaction that NHP 2017 not only validates the earlier critique but the manner in which some malevolent changes have been incorporated in it further strengthen the reasons for our concerns expressed earlier. A nuanced response to the new policy document demands a careful look at these changes made to the draft policy. However, the spirit of a constructive criticism obligates that we begin by registering our appreciation for the policy where it is due. It may also be stated that this postscript shall avoid repeating the arguments made in the earlier critique except for the expediency of aaspect being emphasized afresh.

Credit is due to the policy makers for reaffirming the objective to:

> *'Improve health status through concerted policy action in all sectors and expand preventive, promotive, curative, palliative and rehabilitative services provided through the public health sector with focus on quality'* (emphasis ours) (MOHFW, 2017 a, 3).

Laudably the policy also resolves to raise the public expenditure on health to up to 2.5 per cent of the GDP in order to facilitate this objective and it shall be preferred to raise these funds through general taxation (MOHFW, 2017 a, 5).

We couldn't possibly ask for more than for these solemn commitments to come true. But in the real world it is always wise for our aspirations to be minded by realpolitik. Such promises are nothing new and have been failed repeatedly. The resolve of the

United Progressive Alliance (UPA) Government to raise public expenditure on health to three per cent of the GDP while it rolled out NRHM (National Rural Health Mission) from 2005 to 2011 couldn't fructify. The present Modi government nipped the possibility of such a blasphemy being committed against public exchequer by an affectless slashing of health budget by 20 per cent in the very first budget presented by the government in 2014. Lest our aspirations be more stubborn, Arvind Pangaria, the vice-chairperson of NITI (National Institution for Transforming India) Aayog, Planning Commission's successor body, finds three quarters of a per cent of GDP to be enough to take care of the health needs of India's poor (Panagaria, 2014 quoted in Kurian, 2015). It is fascinating that the kind concerns of India's rulers for their poorer countrymen seem to be waning at a time when our economy is ostensibly pacing ahead of the rest in the world. But 'hope'has a tough soul. Even though the circumstances remain daunting, one needn't lose hope.

The most appreciable and bold aspect of this policy document is the adoption of 'Specific Quantitative Goals and Objectives.' It is stated:

> The indicative, quantitative goals and objectives are outlined under three broad components viz. (a) health status and programme impact, (b) health systems performance and (c) health system strengthening. These goals and objectives are aligned to achieve sustainable development in health sector in keeping with the policy thrust (MOHFW, 2017 a, 3).

The achievements of this policy shall now be measured against these benchmarks. Indeed these benchmarks shall be held to hold the government and the health establishment accountable with respect to success and failures in improving the health status of Indian people.

What is worrying though is India's track record in measuring up to the benchmarks set in the past. With respect to progress made in achieving the MDGs (Millennium Development Goals) it is stated in the 'Situation Analysis' document of NHP 2017 that:

> India is close to reaching the Millennium Development Goals (MDGs) ...From a baseline of 556 in 1990, the nation has achieved Maternal

> Mortality Ratio (MMR) of 167 by 2011-13. Assuming that the Annual Compound Rate of decline observed during 2007-09 and 2011-13 continues, the MMR is likely to reach the MDG-5 target of 139. In case of under-5 mortality rate (U5MR) the MDG target is 42. From a baseline of 126 in 1990, the nation has reached an U5MR of 49 in 2013, and if the rate of reduction over the past decade is sustained, the achievement in 2015 will be very close to the target (MOHFW, 2017 b, 1).

There is nothing in the document by way of analysis of what facilitated and what hindered the achievement of these goals; resultantly, it is near impossible to configure anything about what might have been achieved towards development of country's public health capacity through the listed achievements; or for that matter what are messages to be learnt from past mistakes if any?

Let us try and put these achievements in perspective. As per headline news carried in the *The Hindu*, and most definitely other newspapers as well, on 19 May, Somalia had surpassed India in ensuring the survival of its newborns (*The Hindu*, 2017). Our presumptuous attitudes towards poorer countries apart, quotinga study published in the journal *The Lancet* the report further informed:

> In the GBD (Global Burden of Disease) rankings for health care access and quality (HAQ), India has fallen 11 places, and now ranks 154 out of 195 countries. Further, India's health care index of 44.8 is the lowest among the sub-continental countries, as Sri Lanka (72.8), Bangladesh (51.7), Bhutan (52.7), and Nepal (50.8) all fared better. ...India's downward slide in the rankings indicates that it has failed to achieve health care targets, especially those concerning neonatal disorders, maternal health, tuberculosis, and rheumatic heart disease. Last year, India was ranked 143 among 188 countries.
>
> In the case of neonatal mortality, on a scale of 1 to 100, India scored 14 in the HAQ index, while Afghanistan scored 19/100 and Somalia, 21/100. Access to tuberculosis treatment in India was scored 26 out of 100, lower than Pakistan (29), Congo (30) and Djibouti (29) (*The Hindu*, 2017).

There was much in that article to leave us worried about the state of health in our country. But of course, these days we are kept busy worrying about the holy cow, the checks on anti-nationalism and what not. Who has time to bother about such flabbergasting anti-national nonsense? Resultantly, this headline was forgotten no sooner than it appeared with much deserved deliberation.

The 'Situation Analysis' document mercifully includes a paragraph on 'Social Determinants of Health.' The salience of this paragraph lies in demonstrating the lacklusterand casual attitude towards public health that has become so typical of the generalist bureaucracy in the corridors of the health ministry. The passage of concern over here goes as follows:

> This policy recognizes the causal links between health outcomes and social determinants of health.[18] Health of the population is determined largely by lifestyle (50%) followed by biological and environmental factors (20% each), whereas health systems related factors contribute only 10%.[19] Achievement of national health goals would require addressing all the social determinants (distal and proximal) in the *context of rapid economic growth and changing life styles* (emphasis ours) with a focus on the most vulnerable and marginalized. This preventive aspect needs to be adequately addressed through assessing the impact of existing and future non-health sector programmes and policies through the health lens (MOHFW, 2017 b).

Our officious mandarins are obviously convinced that they deserve first world company, and thewords *'context ofrapid economic growth and changing life styles'* (emphasis ours) are thrown in to assert this conviction. It should not surprise anyone then that the word poverty does not merit even a passing mention among the social determinants of health despite it being the most important matrix that shapes the health of the hundreds of millions of our working people for whom this policy seeks to make most of the difference. One need be reminded here that the 'National Commission for Employment in Unorganized Sector' (NCEUS) had famously declared that 77 per cent of Indians subsisted on less than Rs 20 aday. Additionally, it took an expenditure of just Rs 96or more per capita per day for a person to graduate to 'High Income Group' (Sengupta, 2008). These figures show the mirror to the much acclaimed success of our economic reforms. This was the situation in 2007. Since the world economic crisis of 2008 the lives of the people, as also the economy have been on a slippery slope despite spirited efforts in make believe by inventing newer ways of calibrating upwardly mobile GDP figures.

The reference 18 in the above refers to a WHO report titled - 'WHO (2008): Closing the gap in a generation: health equity through action on the social determinants of health, Final Report of the Commission on Social Determinants of Health, Geneva.' While this is no doubt an authoritative reference but there is a huge body of literature on the social determinants of health from India, which if referred to would have highlighted that the 'vulnerable and marginalized' is not such and ambiguous entity as it has been made to sound. Just as in the case of United States it is the Blacks and other racial minorities, in India's case it is the oppressed castes, the tribal people and the religious minorities who constitute the distinct social and political groups facing systemic and systematic discrimination leading to their social and political marginalization. It is the fear of recogniton of such a discrimination that has kept the 'vulnerable and marginalized' ambiguous. Besides the acknowledgement of this fact is likely to rub sensibilities of the present government at the centre the wrong way inviting the epithet of being ignominous to 'Bharat Mata' whi[illegible] their eyes is characteristic of Left leaning intellec[illegible] It may also be specified that as of today, anyone who is even in the least critical of government's policies is being targeted as a Left leaning intellectual in the academia.

In the same passage reference number 19 also deserves special attention. It is - '*U.S. Department of Health and Human Services. Physical Activity and Health: A Report of the Surgeon General. Atlanta, GA: U.S. Department of Health and Human Services, Centers for Disease Control and Prevention, National Center for Chronic Disease Prevention and Health Promotion, 1996*' (emphasis ours). Since this reference pertains specifically to the U.S. it follows therefore that the proportions allocated to 'lifestyle factors' (50 per cent), 'biological factors' (20 per cent), 'environmental factors' (20 per cent) and 'health system related factors' (10 per cent) in shaping the health of the population are strictly applicable to the conditions prevalent in the U.S. While the role of these factors in shaping the health of people in India is undeniable, however, their relative impact on health shall be specific to the overall conditions in India.

By way of clarification, it may be noted that overwhelming population in United States is urban and the mechanization of routine day to day activities is far higher; and not just much lower levels of poverty, unlike in India where poverty line is actually a destitution line, the poverty line in U.S. provides for a much more substantive living standard. Vis a vis the conditions in U.S. in India nearly 70 per cent of the population lives in the villages where levels of mechanization remain abyssimally low and poverty is not just extensive but very deeply entrenched as well. Those of our people who suffer likewise are also the ones who are most hard pressed to maintain any level of a dignified existence by reliance on publically funded social sector policies. By no figment of imagination can it be said that the lifestyles of these Indians is the same as that of the American people, and hence an assertion that lifestyle contributes up to 50 per cent while the health system related factors only to a measely 10 per cent in shaping the health of the impoverished Indian masses would be way off the mark.

May be in the case of U.S. sedentary lifestyles and consumption of energy rich fast foods could well be attributed to a considerable extent for resulting in obesity, diabetes and hypertention; however, lifestyles can hardly explain entirely the epidemic of diabetes that has come to afflict even the poor in India. Barker's hypothesis, that holds intergenerational transmission of the effects of undernutrition by producing compromised development of various organs of the baby in utero as the cause for various chronic diseases in later life provides a much more likely explanation of this epidemic in the Indian context. Taking the case of a daily wage manual laborer living in an urban slum and a landless agricultural laborer, the health system (which by definition is distinct from health services system and encompasses almost the entire development sector), would any day play a much larger role in shaping their health rather than their impoverished lifestyles.

This reference taken from a developed country's context has been cited on purpose rather than being an oversight. Ascribing as high a role as 50 per cent to lifestyle factors places the responsibility of improving their health overwhelmingly on the people themselves. This is to say that individual factors are predominant in shaping of people's health and that the health system can only possibly assist individual efforts. By extention then one could also say that a dysfunctional health system would at its worst affect peoples' health adversely only to the extent of 10 per cent. This conveniently works towards reducing the government's liability in shaping peoples' health. This facilitates a rationale for rolling back of public health care systems and leave the field wide open for privatization of health care services. This is actually is the essesce of NHP 2017 which is presented in a circutous manner amounting to public healh chicanery on part of the health planners.

NHP 2017 carries over from DNHP the laudatory references to high growth rates of the health care industry in the country. Government's being "invested heavily in the last 25 years in building a positive economic climate for the health care industry" is projected as an achievement. These efforts have put paid to in the emergence of a robust private tertiary health care sector.

The DNHP had boldly and forthrightly pulled off the veil of altruism and argued for corporate hospitals to be exempted from the obligation of treating poor paients. It proposed:

> *Given that the private sector operates within the logic of the market and that they contribute to the economy through their contribution to the growth rate and by the national earnings from medical tourism, there need not be any major effort to persuade them to care for the poor* (emphasis ours), as long as their requirements and perceptions do not influence public policy towards universal health care. Where corporate hospitals and medical tourism earnings are through a high degree of associated *hospitality arrangements* (emphasis ours), one could consider forms of taxation/cess, especially for *certain procedures and services*(emphasis ours) as a form of resource mobilization towards the health sector (MOHFW, 2014, 36).

NHP 2017 again seeks to infuse, howsoever clumsily, a sense of altruism with regard to the profit oriented corporate hospitals. The above formulation has been modified thus:

> The policy enunciates the core principle of societal obligation on the part of private institutions to be followed. This would include:
>
> o Operationalization of mechanisms for referral from public health system to charitable hospitals.
>
> o Ensuring that deserving patients can be admitted on designated free/subsidized beds.
>
> The policy proposes to consider forms of resource generation, where corporate hospitals and medical tourism earnings are through a high

> degree of associated *hospitality arrangements* (emphasis ours) and on account of *certain procedures and services* (emphasis ours), as a form of resource mobilization towards the health sector (MOHFW, 2017 a, 15).

This amounts to being wise by the half. In the midst of consecrating revenue generation through *'hospitality arrangements'* and through *'certain procedures and services'* (read unnecessary procedures and services), what is left unexplained is how the two diametrically opposite aims of providing health care to the peple irrespective of their ability to pay and the compulsion for the corporate hospitals for maximizing profit can be reconciled? It would have served well to showcase the confidence that the health policy planners repose in the prescription they propose if even one example had been cited where selfless service to humanity has prospered under the wings of ravening market nihilism. The DNHP at least acknowledged that:

> Though there is an obligation imposed by their access to considerable tax exemptions and public acquisition of land, - it is only a rare private commercially run hospital that meets these obligations*. A number of not for profit hospitals however offer this, but these are few (MOHFW, 2014, 36).
>
> *(those towards fulfillment of public health objectives)

Both the 'Situation Analysis' document for NHP 2017 as also the policy document have been sanitized of this rare acknowledgement without trace from.

The argument that has nevertheless been persisted with is that the government shall turn into a net purchaser of the expertise of these private tertiay hospitals and thereby obviating the need for people to worry on count of affordability. To this it need be stated emphatically that we are no more in the realm of ambiguity with respect to the publically funded health insurance schemes. The experience also has been that reliance on private sector leads to rendering the public sector health care withered and effete. The utter failure of these schemes in achieving their stated objectives after years of their implementation is now attested to by a wealth of evidence from both within the country and from around the world (Reddy K S et.al., 2011; Shukla et.al., 2011; Reddy, 2013; Prasad and Raghavendra, 2012; Mohanan et.al., 2014; Reddy and

Mary, 2013; Selvaraj and Karan, 2012; Narasimhan et.al., 2014; Sujatha Rao, 2014; Averill and Marriott, 2013; Bajpai and Saraya, 2012)

The following statement by David Sanders caps the experience with public health insurance companies with remarkable precision:

> Universal Health Coverage (UHC) is being widely promoted as a panacea for health inequities yet there are fundamental differences in its interpretation and implementation especially on financing. ...health insurance schemes, often promoted by the World Bank and other donors, invariably disadvantage the poorest and unhealthiest. Without more equitable, tax based approaches, inequalities in health will continue to grow and threaten us all.
>
> Professor David Sanders
> Emeritus Professor
> School of Public Health
> University of the Western Cape
> (Quoted in Averill and Marriott, 2013)

The stand alone capability of a robust public health care sector to render curative healhcare to a large section of the population is the only guarantee of government being able to regulate the prices of the health care services being purchased from private sector. Conversely the inability of the government to be able to provide these services due to a wilted public sector healhcare only begets a helpless dependence on private health care sector. Such a situation can lead to two kinds of consequences, one, that the public exchequer is heavily peanalized, and second, that the government simply abdicates its responsibility leading the people to either being unable to access health care or to spiralling out of pocket expenses on health which incidentally was touted as the primary reason for these schemes to come in force.

Even though the policy talks of "Purchasing care after due diligence from non-Government hospitals as a short term strategy *till public systems are strengthened*" (emphasis ours), it would be wiser to be guided by the government's deeds rather than its nebulous promises. The concerted efforts of all the governments since 1990 are responsible for bringing into existence this behemoth of 'Private Health care Industry' and the problems thereof with the corporate tertiary care hospitals at its head. During these past 26 years there have been committees, court cases and investigations which havedocumented umpteen instances of mandatory obligations towards poor patients being brazenly thrown out of the door by corporate hospitals, but one is at a loss to recall even a single instance of any of these hospitals being taken to task for such thuggery having cornered huge public subsidies. Afterall these hospitals are government's babies and the government's commitment to privileging their interest is absolute. Public sector on the other hand is an orphaned baby.

Privileging private sector is also flowing over to other sectors impacting on health, nutrition being one such sector. Malnutrition, both its extent and depth, is one public health problem that has been a blot on India's reputation internationally where we have been humbled by far poorer countries. Unlike DNHP which almost entirely sidelined the subject, NHP 2017 has included a separate section on malnutrition - "Interventions to Address Malnutrition and Micronutrient Deficiencies."

Before we can dwell on the treatment of malnutrition in the policy document some clarificatory facts need be noted by the readers. Perhaps with the only exception of Antarctica, the human race has inhabited almost every corner on earth and so long as people living even in as harsh and sparse an environoment as the Polar regions and the Kalahari Desert in southern Africa, have had enough of their staple food to eat, they have managed to get dietary energy and nutrients, including micrinutrients, to keep themselves healthy (Kuhnleinand Receveur, 1996; Lang, 2014). It would be patently unreasonable for anyone to argue that all Eskimos or Bushmen of Kalahari are malnourished. Nonetheless, any people living on any part of the globe shall suffer from lower dietary energy intakes derived from macronutrients (carbohydrates, fats and proteins) as also a deficiency of micronutrients (vitamins and minerals) due to intake of less than optimal amount of their staple diets. Vitamin B12, which is available only from animal sourcd food, and iron are the only two micronutrients that may occur despite sufficiency of dietary energy and other micronutrients; as to the rest, micronutrient deficiency seldom occurs as a stand alone phenomenon (Kennedy et. al., 2003; Black, 2003) Additionally, poverty is the foremost cause of dietary energy deficiency worldwide.

However, formulation of the problem of malnutrition in NHP 2017 almost puts all these fundamentals on their head. The policy states:

> Malnutrition, especially micronutrient deficiencies, restricts survival, growth and development of children. It contributes to morbidity and mortality in vulnerable population, resulting in substantial diminution in productive capacity in adulthood and consequent reduction in the nation's economic growth and well-being. Recognising this, the policy declares that micronutrient deficiencies would be addressed through a well-planned strategy on micronutrient interventions. Focus would be on reducing micronutrient malnourishment and augmenting initiatives like micro nutrient supplementation, food fortification, screening for anemia and public awareness. ……Policy recommends exploring fortified food and micronutrient sprinkles for addressing deficiencies through Anganwadi centers andschools (MOHFW, 2017 a, 11).

So the problem of malnutrition in India is the problem of micronutrient deficiencies in the main. The enormous amounts of chronic and acute hunger, which result in a high proportion of stunting and underweight (low weight for height) in Indian children have simply gone missing in this narrative. If hunger is erased from the narrative then poverty as the biggest cause of hunger gets knocked out as a bonus. Hence to solve the massive problem of malnutrition in the country we are left with a prescription of micronutrient sprinklers and fortified foods, products which are beyond the capacity of the people to produce by themselves; however, people can certainly produce all manner of food to tackle their hunger provided the state facilitates it with the right policy instruments. There are no awards for guessing that the pharmaceutical companies shall come out as the winners given the solutions being suggested.

Alternatively, the readers are invited to ponder over what could be achieved for health and nutrition, as also for the prosperity of the country, if the government were to launch instead, poverty alleviation programs with land reforms at their core, accompanied with other agrarian reforms in the countryside, while creating sustainable livelihoods for the urban poor. But of course to empower the poor with such measures shall entail disempowering the dominant classes. In the least any sincere effort at poverty reduction and local solutions at making sufficient food available for the people by enlisting their participation would have given agency to the people in an attempt to bette their lot themselves rather than be passive recipients of technological silver bullets controlled by corporations. A people centric solution to the problem of malnutrition would any day stand a much better chance at increasing economic productivity in comparison to the solution suggested in the policy. Additionally, the approaches suggested by the author would have facilitated a far more meaningful intersectoral coordination and viewing of non-health sectors with a health lens as has been laudatorialy referred to in the policy.

The prescriptions of this policy amount to nothing less than a 'Public Health Chicanery.' It is time that we as people we learn to call a spade a spade in order to move away from illusions and towards real solutions. The critique of DNHP also presented here termed the draft policy to be pursuing "an economic agenda in health care policy rather than a public health agenda." The final policy document takes this to the next level which enables us to confidently state that 'the economic agenda is the corporate agenda in health' and this policy fastens us tighter to this agenda.The declaration of National Health Policy 2017 has made the task of achieving 'Health for All' all the more formidable. This forces the health policy on to the agenda of the struggle for the liberation of our people from oppression.

REFERENCES

Averill C and Anna Marriott (2013): 'Universal Health Coverage: Why health insurance schemes are leaving the poor behind.' Oxfam GB for Oxfam International, Oxford, October.

Bajpai V and Anoop Saraya (2012): 'Rashtriya Swasthya Beema Yojana – A Public Health Perspective.' *Indian Journal of Social Work*, Vol. 73(2): 265-286.

Black M M (2003): 'Micronutrient Deficiencies and Cognitive Functioning.' *Journal of Nutrition*, Vol. 133 (11 Suppl 2): 3927S–3931S.

Kuhnlein H V and Olivier Receveur (1996): 'Dietary Change and Traditional Food Systems of Indigenous Peoples.' *Annu Rev. Nuw*, Vol. 16: 417–42.

Kennedy G, G Nantel and P. Shetty (2003): 'The scourge of hidden hunger:

global dimensions of micronutrient deficiencies,' In FAO (2003): *Food, Nutrition and Agriculture*, P Dasgupta and R Hauspi (eds.), Rome. Available from http://www.fao.org/docrep/005/Y8346M/y8346m02.htm on 19 June, 2017.

Lang Ondøej (2014): 'Dietary Adequacy among the native Eskimo.' Bachelor's Diploma Thesis Supervised by Jeffrey Alan Vanderziel, Department of English and American Studies, Faculty of Arts, Masaryk University, Czech Republic.Available from https://is.muni.cz/th/382859/ff_b/BA_Thesis.rtf on 19 June, 2017.

Ministry of Health and Family Welfare (MOHFW) (2017 a): 'National Health Policy 2017.' Government of India, New Delhi.

Ibid., 3.

Ibid., 5.

Ministry of Health and Family Welfare (MOHFW) (2017 b): 'Situation Analysis: Backdrop to the National Health Policy 2017.' Government of India, New Delhi, p. 1.

Ministry of Health and Family Welfare (2014): 'National Health Policy 2015, Draft.' New Delhi, December, 36.

Ministry of Health and Family Welfare (MOHFW) (2017 a): 'National Health Policy 2017.' Government of India, New Delhi, 15.

Mohanan M, Sebastian Bauhoff, Gerard La Forgia, Kimberly Singer Babiarz, Kultar Singhe, Grant Millerf (2014): 'Effect of Chiranjeevi Yojana on institutional deliveries and neonatal and maternal outcomes in Gujarat, India: a difference-in-differences analysis.' Bulletin of World Health Organisation, Vol. 92: 187–194. doi: http://dx.doi.org/10.2471/BLT.13.124644.

Ministry of Health and Family Welfare (MOHFW) (2017 a): 'National Health Policy 2017.' Government of India, New Delhi, 11.

Narasimhan H, V. Boddu, P. Singh, A. Katyal, S. Bergkvist & M. Rao (2014): 'The Best Laid Plans: Access to the Rajiv Aarogyasri community health insurance scheme of Andhra Pradesh.' *Health, Culture and Society*, Vol. 6 (1). DOI 10.5195/hcs.2014.163 | http://hcs.pitt.edu.

Panagariya, Arvind et. al. (2014): *State Level Reforms, Growth, and Development in Indian States, Studies in Indian Economic Policies*, Oxford University Press, New York. Quoted in Kurian O C (2015): 'Financing Health care for all in India: Towards a Common Goal', Oxfam India, May.

Prasad N P and P Raghavendra (2012): 'Health care Models in the Era of Medical Neo-liberalism: A Study of Aarogyasri in Andhra Pradesh.' Economic and Political Weekly, 27 October, Vol. 47 (43): 118 – 126.

Reddy K S, S Selvaraj, K D. Rao, M Chokshi, P Kumar, V Arora and S Bhokare, I Ganguly (2011): 'A Critical Assessment of the Existing

Health Insurance Models in India.' Public Health Foundation of India, New Delhi, 31 January.

Reddy S (2013): 'Aarogyasri Scheme in Andhra Pradesh, India': Some Critical Reflections. *Social Change*, 43(2) 245–261.

Reddy S, Immaculate Mary (2013): 'Rajiv Aarogyasri Community Health Insurance Scheme in Andhra Pradesh, India: A Comprehensive Analytic View of Private Public Partnership Model.' *Indian Journal of Public Health*, October-December, Vol. 57 (4): 254–259.

Sengupta A, K P Kannan, G Raveendran (2008): 'India's Common People: Who Are They, How Many Are They and How Do They Live?' *Economic and Political Weekly*, 15 March; Vol. 43 (11): 49 – 63.

Shukla R, Veena Shatrugna, R Srivatsan (2011): 'Aarogyasri Health care Model: Advantage Private Sector'. *Economic and Political Weekly*, 3 December, Vol. 46 (49): 38 – 42.

Selvaraj S, Anup K Karan (2012): 'Why Publicly-Financed Health Insurance Schemes Are Ineffective in Providing Financial Risk Protection. *Economic and Political Weekly*, Vol. 47 (11): 60 – 68.

Sujatha Rao (2014): 'For public health as political priority.' *The Hindu*, 13 October. Available from http://www.thehindu.com/opinion/lead/for-public-health-as-political-priority/article6493944.ece on 20 October, 2014.

The Hindu (2017): 'Chance of newborn survival: Somalia better off than India', 19 May. Available from http://www.thehindu.com/news/national/chance-of-newborn-survival-somalia-better-off-than-india/article18511050.ece on 17 June, 2017.

6

The Challenges Before Public Hospitals, Their Origins and Possible Solutions

Introduction

Some authors have described large modern-day hospitals as 'monuments to disease'. Indeed, that is what they will remain so long as they function merely as institutions for curative care, detached from the larger social, economic, cultural, and political context of people's lives which is the principal determinant of their health. Unfortunately, even this curative care has become unaffordable to many ordinary people given the policy framework governing India's health sector.

The truth is that public hospitals have become increasingly detached from the larger context in which medicine operates. If public hospitals are to be made responsive to the health needs of the people then the problems afflicting these institutions ought to be viewed within the framework of the broader conditions (we may call these structural problems) that influence their functioning, rather than only within the context of their inner working. This also implies that the solutions to these problems ought to be socially oriented rather than being guided by narrow managerial or techno-centric approaches.

Public sector health care will continue to be relevant for a long time in order to make it available to vast sections of under-served populations in developing countries like India. In the context that India's Twelfth Five Year Plan document has rolled out an ambitious scheme to achieve 'Universal Health Care', this chapter focuses on the greatest challenges facing a public hospital: the sources of these challenges and solutions to them. Here, a public hospital will include the most peripheral PHC (primary health centre) to a tertiary care hospital in a large city.

Even though there are differences in the specific functions of these institutions, yet they constitute a continuum of care, both preventive and curative. While the lower levels ought to provide more direct preventive and curative services for most common diseases, the higher level institutions are supposed to cater to a more select set of patients who are in need of more specialized services not available at the lower public health facilities. Apart from this, the higher public health facilities have an obligation to provide supervision, training, and technical support to facilitate smoother functioning of the primary level facilities. It follows then that there is a synthesis across different levels of public hospitals and a breakdown at any level has consequences for all levels.

Principal Challenges Confronting a Public Hospital

In my view, the principal challenges confronting public hospitals today are:

1. Deficient infrastructure
2. Deficient manpower
3. An unmanageable patient load
4. Equivocal quality of services, and
5. High out-of-pocket expenditure.

Deficient Infrastructure

Figures in parenthesis are the beds per thousand population required to be achieved in the 'Ten Year Plan' and 'Three Million Plan', and the current ratio at in India.

The format of the public health structure in India draws directly from the recommendations of the *Bhore Committee Report, 1946*. However, the public health infrastructure that has evolved lags far behind the content and the spirit of the Committee's Report. The Committee proposed the implementation of its recommendations in two distinct phases: 'three million plan' and the 'ten year plan'.

The 'Three Million Plan' set out the necessary health infrastructure required to meet the health needs of an average district in India with a population of three million. This was to be

Table 1: Comparison Between the 'Ten Year Plan', the 'Three Million Plan' and the Currently Available Health Infrastructure

	'Ten Year Plan' (targets to be met at the end of ten years)			*'Three Million Plan'*			*Present Available Infrastructure*		
	Population Norm	*Medical Officers*	*Hospital*	*Population Norm*	*Medical Officers*	*Hospital*	*Population per Facility*	*Medical Officers*	*Hospital Bed Norms*##
Primary Unit	40,000	2	15 beds	20,000 population	6	75 beds	34,641.3**	1.2	4 beds
Secondary Unit	5,00,000	17	200 beds	6,00,000 population	140	650 beds	1,72,375**	3.3	30
District Headquarters/ Larger Secondary Units	7,50,000	-	500 beds* (1.03/1,000)	30,00,000 population	268	2,500 beds (5.67/1,000)	17,45,152 approx.#	-	100 to 500 beds(.9/1,000)

Note: The 'Three Million Plan' set out the health infrastructure required to provide for the health needs of an average district in India with a population of three million. This was to be implemented over a period of three or four decades. Anticipating resource constraints, both in terms of manpower and finance to make such an infrastructure available over a short period, the Committee recommended a shorter 'ten-year plan' to be implemented first.

Source: Details of the 'Ten Years Plan' and 'Three Million Plan' have been obtained from Chapters III and IV of the Government of India (1946): *Report of the Health Development and Survey Committee (Bhore Committee),* Vol. II, (Government of India Press).

* In the 'Ten Year Plan', the Bhore Committee did not recommend setting up a district-level tertiary health establishment. Instead, 4 of the 200 bed secondary units in the districts were to be elevated to the level 500 of bed secondary units.

**Figures obtained from Table 11 of the *Rural Health Bulletin, 2012* (Ministry of Health and Family Welfare, Government of India [GOI, 2013]).

#The figure has been obtained by dividing India's total population in 2011 by the number of district hospitals.

Obtained from *Rural Health Bulletin, 2012,* (Ministry of Health and Family Welfare [GOI, 2013]).

implemented over a period of three to four decades. Anticipating resource constraints, both in terms of manpower and resources to set up such an infrastructure over a short time, the Committee recommended a shorter 'Ten Year Plan' to be implemented first. Table 1 provides a comparison of the 'Ten Year Plan', 'Three Million Plan', and the public health infrastructure currently available in India.

As against the 0.24 beds per 1,000 population that were available in British India, the Committee's overall plan for development of health services in India provided for establishing 1.03 beds per 1000 population within ten years of implementation of the plan and a ratio of 5.67 beds/1,000 population in 30 to 40 years. The Committee further stated that:

> We consider moreover, that our recommendations constitute an irreducible minimum, and were it not for the limitation imposed by the inadequacy of staff and funds; we should unhesitatingly have proposed a more comprehensive scheme than the one indicated (GOI, 1946, Vol. II, p. 31).

However, even a cursory look at Table 1 indicates that what was considered to be an 'irreducible minimum' by the Committee proved to be a formidable task for achievement by the Indian health planners.

The UPA (United Progressive Alliance) Government launched the ambitious National Rural Health Mission (NRHM) in 2005 to bolster the rural health infrastructure. After completion of the first phase in 2012 the mission is now in the second phase of its implementation. To begin with, the mission was meant to bring the EAG (Empowered Action Group) states which lagged far behind the rest of India in health infrastructure, at par with the rest of the country. Table 2 provides the rural infrastructure status in the EAG states (Jammu & Kashmir and Himachal Pradesh excluded) as on March 2012.

It is clearly evident from the Table that the average shortfall for different types of facilities is between two to three times higher in EAG states as in the non-EAG ones. Similarly, the average population served per facility continues to remain much higher for EAG states as for those for non-EAG states. With the notable

Table 2: Shortfall in Health Infrastructure as on March 2012 in EAG States According to the 2011 Population Census (Provisional) Norms

State	*Sub-Centres (SC)*				*PHCs*				*CHCs*			
	Req.	*In pos.*	*% short.*	*Pop/SC*	*Req.*	*In pos.*	*% short.*	*Pop/PHC*	*Req.*	*In pos.*	*% short.*	*Pop/CHC*
Bihar	18,533	9,696	48%	9,496	3,083	1,863	40%	49,423	770	70	91%	13,15,357
Chhattisgarh	4,904	5,111	-4.2%	3,836	776	755	3%	25,965	194	149	23%	1,31,568
Jharkhand	6,043	3,958	35%	6,326	964	330	66%	75,870	241	188	22%	1,33,175
Madhya Pradesh	12,314	8,869	28%	5,924	1,977	1,156	42%	45,448	494	333	33%	1,57,771
Odisha	8,136	6,688	18%	5,226	1,308	1,226	6%	28,508	327	377	15%	92,709
Rajasthan	15,172	11,487	24%	4,487	2,326	1,528	34%	33,731	581	382	34%	1,34,922
Uttar Pradesh	31,037	20,521	34%	7,559	5,172	3,692	29%	42,013	1,293	515	60%	3,01,186
Uttarakhand	2,341	1,848	21%	3,802	351	257	26.8%	27,337	87	59	32%	1,19,078
EAG states combined	98,480	68,178	30.8%	6,423	15,957	10,807	32.3%	40,518	3,987	2,073	48%	2,11,231
All India – EAG	90,614	80,188	11.5%	4,928	14,608	13,242	9.4%	29,845	3,644	2,760	24.3%	1,43,191
All India	189,094	1,48,366	23%	5,615	30,565	24,049	26%	34,641	7,631	4,833	40%	1,72,375

Source: All figures are taken/calculated on the basis of figures in Table 11, *RHS Bulletin*, 2012, MOHFW, GOI [GOI, 2013].

exceptions of Chhattisgarh, Odisha, Uttarakhand, and Jharkhand for the number of CHCs in position, the shortfall for different levels of facilities in the other five states is much higher than the all India average.

The relative advantage of states like Chhattisgarh, Odisha, and Uttarakhand may well be illusory because, as we will see shortly, the mere availability of infrastructure does not mean it is delivering the required services, which along with infrastructure also depend on the availability of amenities such as water, electricity, beds, medical and paramedical manpower, and spatial distribution of the available infrastructure. Table 3 illustrates some of the other deficiencies of the available infrastructure which undermines its functional status.

Table 3: Some of the Deficiencies in the Available Infrastructure

Indicator	*Shortfall (percentage)*
Sub-centres without ANM	3.2
PHCs without doctor	3.8
Sub-centres without regular water supply	25.5
Sub-centres without electric supply	25.5
Sub-centres without all whether motor able roads	6.6
PHCs without regular electric supply	8
PHCs without regular water supply	10.7
PHCs without all-weather motor-able roads	5.8

Source: *RHS Bulletin*, 2012, MOHFW (GOI, 2013).

Non-availability of facilities such as water and electricity can only be expected to deeply undermine the functioning of existing facilities. It is extremely possible that if the facility has one resource it may lack other resources to optimally use the available resources, for example, if a health worker is available at the facility, it may not have water/electricity, thus undermining the ability of the health worker to perform his/her functions optimally.

A mismatch in the spatial distribution of infrastructure is another factor that magnifies the deficiency of infrastructure. Fig. 1 illustrates this aspect very well. One can clearly see that there is a concentration of available beds in a tiny proportion of the larger cities. If the same beds were to be more equitably distributed

Fig. 1: Distribution of Available Hospital Beds in India

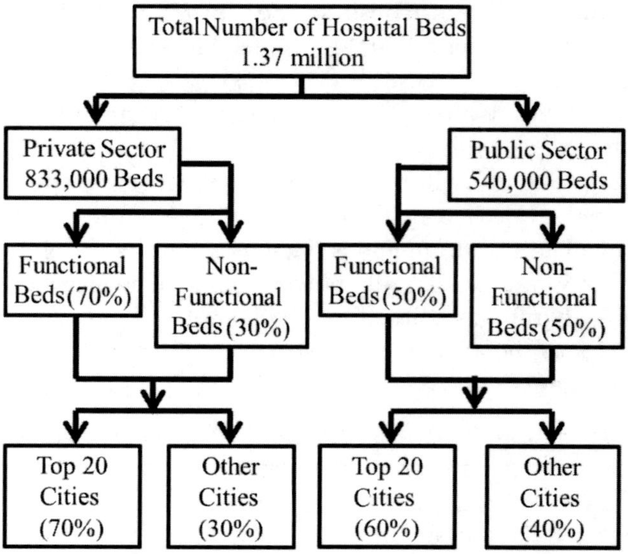

Source: Mehta et al., 2010.

between cities and between urban and rural areas, availability of the same infrastructure would have gone a longer way in ameliorating the curative needs of the people. However, such a situation is the logical outcome of the development paradigm pursued in India rather than an inadvertent occurrence.

A comparison of the availability of hospital beds per 1,000 population between India and some much poorer countries (Table 4) offers a telling comment on the sufficiency of India's health infrastructure. Many sub-Saharan countries and a country as impoverished as Timor-Leste seem to be faring far better.

Table 4: A Comparison of Availability of Hospital Beds for Selected Countries

Country	*Timor-Leste*	*Gabon*	*Equatorial Guinea*	*Djibouti*	*Kenya*	*Botswana*	*Zambia*	*India*
Beds/ 1,000 population	5.9	6.3	2.1	1.4	1.4	1.8	2	.9

Source: World Development Indicators, World Bank Data Bank.

Deficient Manpower

Deficiency of human resources in health is a serious additional problem to that of a deficiency in health infrastructure. Deficiency of human resources in health occurs at several levels: between regions, between rural and urban areas, and between the public and private sector. On one hand there is an unwillingness of doctors and other health personnel to serve in rural areas, on the other, even in the urban areas there is a preponderance of the health manpower in the dominant, for profit, private health sector in India, thereby putting their services beyond the reach of the majority of poor in the country.

The deficiency of specialists in rural health care is as high as over 90 per cent in Chhattisgarh, Odisha, and Rajasthan, while being at a high of nearly 85 per cent in Uttarakhand. The inter-regional disparities are also explicit with there being a wide gap in the deficiency of both specialist and graduate doctors between the EAG and the non-EAG states. Even though there appears to be an excess of GDMOs in Bihar and a relatively smaller shortfall in Jharkhand as against the required posts, this is highly misleading as the overall physicians per 10,000 population ratio remains dismal at 0.5 for both the states. The 'required' here signifies required as against the sanctioned posts and not the requirement vis-à-vis some population norm. For example, the total rural population of Bihar was 92.07 million according to the 2011 Census, whereas the total number of doctors required (specialists and GDMOs) in the rural health set-up, according to Table 5 is only 2,773. This would amount to only 0.3 doctors per 10,000 rural population which is a travesty of any norm. Even after seven years of implementation of the NRHM (National Rural Health Mission) there remain a wide gap in the availability of allopathic doctors in the rural areas between the non-EAG states and EAG states; in the former 2.25 times more.

Notwithstanding deficiencies in their training as managerial physicians, doctors have generally come to be perceived as responsible members of the health care team comprising paramedical and other support staff. They are expected to lead the way in problem solving and supervising the work of other team members. As such, the deficiency of doctors, besides impacting

Table 5: The Number of Specialists and MBBS Doctors Serving in Public Sector Rural Health care in the EAG States, Non-EAG States, and All-India

State	*CHCs*				*PHCs*		*Total GDMOs*		*Shortfall*		*Physicians per 10,000 Rural Population*
	Specialists		*GDMOs*		*GDMOs*				*Specialists*	*GDMOs*	
	Req.	*In pos.*	*Req.*	*In pos.*	*Req.*	*In pos.*	*Req.*	*In pos.*	*%*	*%*	
Bihar	420	151	490	451	1863	3532	2353	3983	64%	-69.3%	0.5
Chhattisgarh	894	71	1043	347	755	435	1798	782	92%	56.5%	0.4
Jharkhand	1128	86	1316	757	330	407	1646	1164	92.4%	29.3%	0.5
Madhya Pradesh	1998	267	2331	678	1156	814	3487	1492	86.6%	57.2%	0.3
Odisha	2262	317	2639	278	1226	1069	3865	1347	86%	65.15%	0.5
Rajasthan	2292	148	2674	265	1528	1755	4202	2020	93.5%	51.9%	0.4
Uttar Pradesh	3090	1740	3605	167	3692	2861	7297	3028	43.7%	58.5%	0.3
Uttarakhand	354	51	413	40	257	205	670	245	85.6%	63.4%	0.4
EAG States Total	12438	2831	14511	2983	10807	11078	25318	14061	77.2%	44.5%	0.4
Non-EAG States	6894	3027	19320	6928	13242	17906	32562	24834	56.1%	23.7%	0.09
All India	19332	5858	33831	9911	24049	28984	57880	38895	69.7%	32.8%	0.06

Source: Based on data taken from *RHS Bulletin*, 2012 [GOI, 2013]. Note: GDMO = General Duty Medical Officer.

the delivery of curative services, may also reflect adversely in the overall functioning of the health team.

Figure 2: Shortfall in Various Categories of Paramedical Staff in the Rural Health care Set Up, All-India.

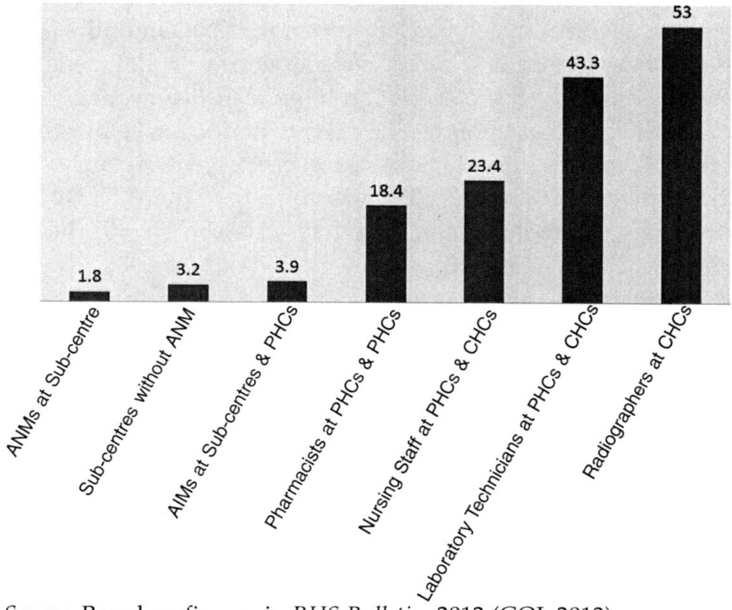

Source: Based on figures in *RHS Bulletin*, 2012 (GOI, 2013).

Deficiency of health personnel is by no means limited to doctors alone. Fig. 2 illustrates the shortfall in various categories of paramedical personnel in the public sector rural health care system. It may be pointed here that some countries such as the Soviet Union in the immediate aftermath of the Bolshevik Revolution and China, made up for the deficiency in strength of doctors by training and deploying a huge cadre of paramedical public health personnel in the poorly served areas.

The shortage of manpower is only aggravated by the absence of a comprehensive and integrated health manpower policy dealing with the requirement projection of health manpower, manpower production, training, recruitment, career development, supportive supervision, skill enhancement, postings in under-served areas, retention and transfers, etc (Nandan, D., et al., 2007; Rao, et al.,

2011). This remains the case notwithstanding a number of official committees having stressed the need for a comprehensive health health manpower policy beginning with the *Bhore Committee Report* of 1946 itself (HLEG, 2011).

The skewed distribution of the available health cadre of different categories which has left the rural, tribal, and hilly areas grossly underserved is a direct consequence of a deficiency in human resources and the lack of an integrated health manpower resource development policy. The density of doctors is four times and that of nurses is three times higher in urban areas in comparison to the rural areas (Rao et al., 2009). According to the WHO, of the 57 countries facing a Human Resources crisis in Health, India's ranking is 52nd (WHO, 2010).

Statistics per se alone may still not give a complete idea of the acuteness of the challenge as perhaps can a description of the ground realities. While working as a consultant at the National Health Services Resource Centre (NHSRC), I had the opportunity to visit many health facilities in different districts of Uttar Pradesh and Uttarakhand. The following are observations from some of the visits:

- During a monitoring visit I made in June 2013 to the district hospital in Pithoragarh district of Uttarakhand state I found that the doctors and the employees were on strike in protest against the roughing up of some hospital staff by the relatives of a 18 or 19-year-old boy who had died the previous night of some complication following an operation for abdominal/inguinal hernia (a simple and routine procedure provided there is no strangulation of the intestines at the site of the hernia).

  At the time the boy died there were only two nurses, one in the casualty ward of the hospital and the other caring for the patients who had been admitted to the various wards, in the 120-bed hospital. After the regular working hours there is only one doctor available for all these patients and that too in the emergency ward. Therefore, in the absence of doctors and nurses in the wards after normal hours, it is for the attendants to be able to locate them in the hospital in the event of their patient requiring medical attention, provided of course the attendants are able to judge the criticality of their patients' discomfort.

- Similarly, in the 100-bed District Women's Hospital at Jhansi after 4 pm there is only one nurse (who was working on contract basis at the time of my visit) to attend to the labour room, the ward, and an occasional Cesarean section that might be required. A hundred beds do not mean only a hundred patients for one need also to count the babies of the mothers who have delivered.
- The conditions at the 100-bed Mahatma Gandhi Smarak District Hospital at Naugarh, the district headquarter of Siddharthnagar district in UP are even worse. The patients are pretty much on their own after 4 pm as the only available nurse is kept busy in the labour room, while the doctor mans the emergency. The hospital had just 5 nurses on its rolls at the time of writing to provide all the nursing care required at the hospital.
- Almost similar conditions were prevalent at the District General and the District Women's Hospital in Faizabad district of Uttar Pradesh. According to the information provided by the hospital authorities in February 2013, there had been 26 maternal deaths at the hospital over the past year out of a total of 5,860 deliveries. This works out to a maternal mortality rate of a whopping 443.7 per 100,000 live births.
- There was just one obstetrician and gynecologist in both Pithoragarh and Siddharthnagar districts to cater to cases requiring Cesarean deliveries. The specialist in Pithoragarh lived around 580 kms away from her family in Gwalior, situated in Madhya Pradesh state. She was forthright: 'Had I been posted in the plain areas I could have at least visited my family easily. I am only biding my time and shall leave the moment I get a more suitable job.'

Given such conditions, it should be no surprise that crucial hospital procedures such as maintaining sterilization practices in the operation theatres, labour rooms, newborn-care units, and intensive care units are simply given a go by or are so done that leaves much to be desired. This cannot but have a negative impact on the morale of the health workers. The medical officer in charge of the CHC at Baijnath in Bageshwar district, Uttarakhand, lamented: 'Given the patient load and strength of doctors at my facility I am hardly able to give a minute per patient in the OPD; this makes me wonder about the worth of my work; what quality of services are we providing?'

Unmanageable Patient Load

Secondary or tertiary level public hospitals in the larger cities are today bursting at the seams due to the heavy rush of patients. The huge unplanned increase in the size of Indian cities has resulted in the urbanization of rural poverty causing expansion of slums and marginal populations starved of health and other basic amenities. The deficiency of the urban health infrastructure, overcrowding in hospitals, lack of outreach and a functional referral system, standards and norms for the urban health care delivery system, social exclusion, unavailability or ignorance of information on how to access modern health care facilities, and lack of purchasing power are some of the issues that have been identified as challenges to urban health care in India (John et al., 2008). These factors are further complicated by poorly functioning sub-centres, PHCs, and CHCs, resulting in people from rural areas having to increasingly depend on hospitals in the larger cities and towns for their curative needs and thereby stretching beyond their limits the infrastructure at these hospitals. Some idea of the level of functioning of the peripheral health facilities in India is provided in Table 6 below.

The problems reflected in Table 6 are further accentuated by high rates of absenteeism among health workers. According to a nationally representative all-India survey conducted in 2003, nearly 40 per cent of the doctors and other health service providers were found to be absent from their posts on a typical working day. While absenteeism among doctors varied between 30 per cent in Madhya Pradesh to 67 per cent in Bihar (the figure on availability of GDMOs, given in Table 5, in excess of requirement should be viewed in this context); it was found to be 30 per cent among pharmacists and laboratory technicians (Muralidharan, 2011).

Table 6: Deficiencies in Functioning of PHCs and CHCs in India

Primary Health Centres (Percentage)	
PHCs without residential quarter for medical officer	45.5
PHCs that did not provide 24 hour services	47.3
PHCs conducting less than 10 normal deliveries a month	50
Community Health Centres (Percentage)	
CHCs not performing even normal delivery services	10
CHC not designated as First Referral Units (FRUs)	48
CHCs functioning without an obstetrician/gynecologist	74.8
CHCs without a functional operation theatre	34.8
FRUs with blood storage facilities	9.1
FRUs without 24 hour new born care facilities	23.9

Source: GOI, 2010.

Note: These statistics relate to a time when the NRHM began; there may have been marginal improvements over the period after the implementation of the NRHM but comparable national level statistics for a later period are not available. Anyhow, it is nobody's claim that the implementation of the NRHM has reduced the workload on public health facilities in the larger urban centres, especially as almost the entire focus of the NRHM has been improvement in the maternal and child health services and also on improving the rates of institutional deliveries with the objective of reducing maternal and infant mortality. Unfortunately, even the delivery of these services remains far from desirable and of desirable quality.

The pattern of organization of the health services into primary, secondary, and tertiary levels implies a referral system between these levels such that the patients who cannot be handled at the primary or secondary levels can be referred to the higher levels for appropriate management. A referral system does not however imply exclusivity between different levels of health care. Rather, it entails active cooperation between them that is necessary for the development of the health services system as a whole. In this context the *Bhore Committee Report* states:

> The heads of different sections in the district hospitals dealing with medicine, surgery and so on ...it will be of advantage if they can occasionally visit the secondary unit hospitals and a certain number of primary unit hospitals and inspect and guide the professional work of officers discharging corresponding duties in these hospitals. Such contacts should help to improve the standard of professional work carried out in the hospitals of the districts generally.' (GOI, 1946, Vol. II, p. 21).

Apart from this, the Committee also laid stress on the need for the tertiary level hospitals to play a role in the training and continuing skill enhancement for different categories of health personnel (Ibid., p. 22).

Contrary to this, there is barely a 'referral system' worth its name that operates in the Indian public health set-up. Rather, the poor functioning or even the absence of the peripheral health services in large parts leaves patients with no alternative but to throng to the already overstretched facilities of larger hospitals in towns and cities, causing a marked deterioration in their functioning.

A study conducted at three referral hospitals in Lucknow district showed that nearly 90 per cent of the patients coming to them were new patients, and of these two-thirds had reached directly without any referral. Overall, only around a tenth of all patients attending these hospital had been referred by someone, while the rest were all self-referred (Bhola et al., 2008).

This trend is further aggravated by some of the policy prescriptions of the government. For example, during a field visit to one of the 'Empowered Group States' of north India by me, the principal secretary health of the state in a meeting acknowledged the immense pressure on the largest public hospital in the capital of the state on account of the 'Janani Suraksha Yojana', an institutional delivery scheme, under the NRHM sponsored by the central government to reduce the rates of maternal mortality and the neo-natal mortality. The non-functioning or under-performance of the peripheral health institutions as delivery points and the assistance of a government-sponsored ambulance service, there had caused such a rush of maternity cases to the hospital that the doctors pleaded: 'For God's sake, halt this madness.' Another fall-out of this has been that the ambulance service sponsored by the state has established a world record in 'deliveries conducted on the way' to hospital.

While there has been a certain decline in maternal and infant mortality rates due to this scheme is, it has certainly stretched the services of the state's tertiary health care services well beyond capacity.

Equivocal Quality of Services

A patient load far in excess of what the infrastructure is capable of handling is bound to undermine the quality of care. 'Chacha Nehru Bal Chikitsalaya', a Delhi government run child care hospital in east Delhi had much to celebrate when it became the first public hospital in the capital to be accredited by the National Accreditation Board for Hospitals (NABH). However, with the patient load bursting at the seams, the hospital soon found itself struggling to survive. The resources for the very essential expansion of infrastructure to cope with the rush of patients have been difficult to come by (Chandra, N., 2012).

Figure 3: Inpatient and Outpatient Share of Public Hospitals in Rural and Urban Areas

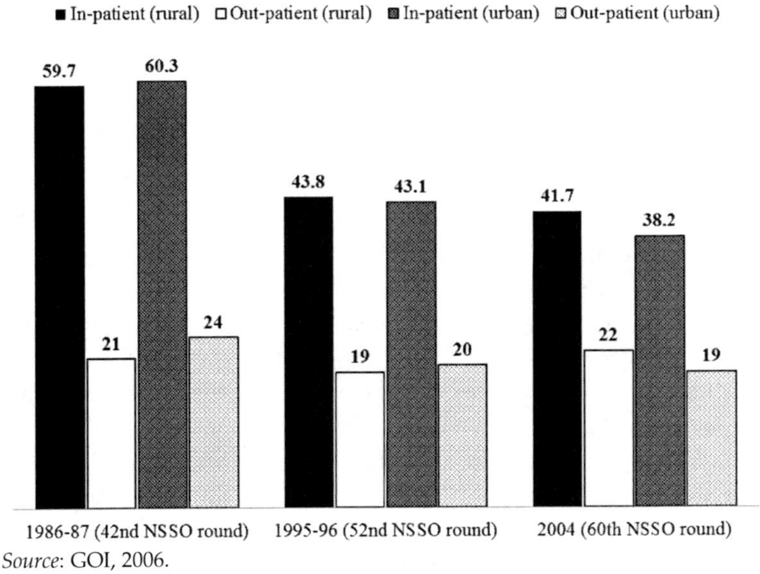

Source: GOI, 2006.

Apart from general deficiencies in the development of public health infrastructure in India, there has been a particularly marked deterioration in the services of public hospitals for over two decades in pursuit of neoliberal policies in general and in health sector too which have been oriented towards strengthening private health-care. The growing dominance of private health care has resulted in the moulding of public hospitals too in the image of private hospitals. Some of the steps taken in this direction have been outsourcing of many services in public hospitals such as security, laundry, cleaning, kitchen services, and, in later stages, even the diagnostic and curative facilities on the public-private partnership model. The progressive imposition of user charges is another such feature (Jan Swasthya Abhiyan, 2006a).

While there is no evidence of these measures having resulted in improvement of the services of public hospitals, there is every reason to believe that these measures have made the services of public hospitals more inaccessible to the common man. Notwithstanding the persistent rush of patients, Fig. 3 shows that the proportionate share of public hospitals in hospitalized care has continued to decrease while it is about stagnant for out-patient care. Apart from this, the private sector has been poaching on the trained manpower of public hospitals (Jha, 2012; Perappadan, 2012) at a considerable cost to the quality of services in public hospitals.

High Out-of-Pocket Expenditure

The last issue of *National Health Accounts for India* published in 2004-5 unambiguously stated: 'Among all the sources, households contributed a significant portion at 71.13 per cent of total health expenditure for availing of health care services from different health care institutions. This covers expenditure on inpatient, outpatient care, family planning, and immunization, etc.' (GOI, 2004–05). Table 7 below gives some health spending patterns for India and her neighbours and some other select countries. The only saving grace for India is that among its neighbours, Pakistan and Myanmar spend less public resources on health than India. India's public expenditure on health fails to match even that of the least developed countries and sub-Saharan Africa.

It is generally acknowledged that catastrophically low health expenditure is a significant cause for people being pushed below the poverty line in India. Table 8 shows that 2.13 per cent more people were pushed below the poverty line on account of out-of-pocket (OOP) expenditure on health between 1993-4 and 2004-5. The decade between 1993-4 and 2004-5 was the period when neoliberal economic reforms were at their zenith. A reading of the data in Tables 8, 9, 10, and 11 cannot but reflect the impact of these

Table 7: Health Spending Indicators for Select Group of Countries, India and Her Neighbours, 2010

Country/Group of Countries	*Health Expenditure Public as % of GDP*	*Private Expenditure on Health as % of Total Expenditure on Health*	*Out-of-pocket Expenditure as % of Private Expenditure on Health*	*Out-of-pocket Expenditure as % of Total Expenditure on Health*
South Asia	1.08	70.9	80.7	61.5
India	1.06	71.8	86.0	61.8
Afghanistan	2.35	77.5	94.0	72.8
Bangladesh	1.35	63.5	96.6	61.3
Bhutan	3.60	15.4	94.7	14.5
China	2.70	45.7	77.2	35.3
Maldives	3.80	39.2	71.6	28.1
Myanmar	0.24	87.9	92.7	81.5
Nepal	1.89	62.6	90.4	56.6
Pakistan	0.79	71.8	88.0	63.2
Sri Lanka	1.57	54.4	81.9	44.6
Cuba	9.70	4.8	100	4.8
USA	8.49	51.8	22.7	11.8
OECD countries	7.94	37.4	-	-
Lower middle income countries	1.51	64.6	85.8	56.4
Low income countries	2.11	62.9	75.9	49.6
Least developed countries	2.18	60.9	80.7	50.5
Sub-Saharan Africa (developing countries)	2.8	56.8	62.8	30.9

Source: Health Nutrition and Population Statistics in World Bank Databank. Available from http://databank.worldbank.org/data/views/variableselection/selectvariables. aspx?source=health-nutrition-and-population-statistics and accessed on 15 August 2013.

reforms on the state of the people's health.

During this period there was an increase in OOP expenditure as a proportion of the total household (HH) consumption expenditure across expenditure quintiles. The highest increase was in the 'Richest' quintile; however, before we jump to the conclusion that this was due to greater health.

Table 8: Out-of-Pocket (OOP) Expenditure as a % of Total Household Expenditure and Impoverishment Due to OOP

Year	*Mean OOP as % of total HH expn.*	*Mean OOP as % of total HH expenditure by expenditure quintile*					*% HH having catastrophic exp. @ OOP expen. >10% of total HH exp.*	*% people impoverished due to OOP*
		Poorest	*2nd poorest*	*Middle*	*2nd richest*	*Richest*		
1993-94	4.39	3.25	4.19	4.68	5.23	5.45	15.12%	4.0
2004-05	5.51	4.00	5.01	5.92	6.69	7.09	17.25%	4.4

Source: Ghosh, S., 2010. Note: My cross-sectional data are from the fiftieth (1993–4) and sixty-first (2005) rounds of national and state representative surveys on 'consumption expenditure' collected by the National Sample Survey Organization, India.

Table 9: Average Medical Expenditure (Rs) Per Hospitalization and Non-Hospitalization Case

Type of Hospital	*Expenditure per Hospitalization Case (Rs)*					*Expenditure per Non-Hospitalization Case (Rs)*			
	All India	*Rural*		*Urban*		*Rural*		*Urban*	
	2014*	2004	1995-6	2004	1995-6	2014**	2004	2014**	2004
Government Hospital	6,120	3,238	2,080	3,877	2,195	456	11	391.5	7
Private Hospital	25,850	7,408	4,300	11,553	5,344	791.5	246	958	299
Any Hospital	-	5,695	3,202	8,851	3,921	-	-	-	-

Source: Figures for 1995-6 have been obtained from GOI, 2006, Statements 28 and 32 while figures for 2014 have been obtained from GOI, 2015, Statements 3.9 and 3.15.

Note: *The separate figures for expenditure per hospitalization case in rural and urban areas for the year 2014 were not available. **The figures for 2014 are simple arithmetic mean of average expenditure per non-hospitalization case by gender. A weighted average could not be calculated as the number of men and women contributing to calculation of per man and woman expenditure was not known.

Table 9 makes it evident that both inpatient and outpatient care is much more expensive in the private sector. If we see the findings of Tables 8 and 9 in light of Fig. 3 above, it becomes clear that the increasing share of the private sector in provisioning of health care is to a large extent responsible for increasing OOP expenditure on health. With public health care becoming even more dwarfed by the private sector, the latter has increasingly begun to set the standards both for care and its cost, at terms congenial to its propensity for profit-making. Increasing commercialization of the services of public hospitals through measures such as imposition of user charges at all levels under the impact of the dominant private sector has heightened the challenges facing a public hospital in meeting the people's curative needs. The steep rise in the medical expenditure per person, particularly for non-hospitalization cases in public hospitals between 2004 and 2014 is a case in point.

The Social and Political Origins of the Crisis of the Public Hospital

The present always originates from the womb of the past. In order to understand the origins of the challenges facing a public hospital we need to put things in their historical perspective. We have already referred in Chapter 3 to the famous minute of Thomas Macaulay on education in India delivered on February 2, 1835 in the British parliament, wherein he talks of creating a class of persons in India who are 'Indian in blood and colour, but English in taste, in opinions, in morals, and in intellect" (Macaulay, T.B., 1835).

How well the designs of colonial masters have fructified is epitomized by the following words of our present speech delivered by former Indian Prime Minister, Dr Manmohan Singh, at Oxford (Singh, Manmohan, 2005), which has already been quoted in Chapter 3. The sentiments expressed by Dr Singh were only seconded by his Finance Minister, Mr. P. Chidambaram, when addressing the investors in London in 1997, he said:

> You came to India and stayed for 200 years. Now come prepared to invest and stay for another 200 years and there will be huge rewards (Verma, 1997).

People's long experience of governance over the 65 years since independence attests to the truth of these words. There is much that can be said and demonstrated by highlighting the essentially reactionary character of India's ruling classes towards the overwhelming mass of impoverished Indians. One need not dwell on that here, the intention merely being to point to this reactionary character of the Indian state in relation to the formulation of its development policy.

The very fact that the Indian ruling classes have retained the coercive colonial machinery in letter and in spirit speaks volumes about their sincerity in ensuring the welfare of India's impoverished people. The following passage about the 'Indian Police Act of 1861' illustrates the real meaning of 'Our notions of the rule of law' that Manmohan Singh spoke of at Oxford.

'The Indian Police Act of 1861 was primarily a mechanism to subjugate the people, and the traditional cooperation of the community was lost sight of in the concerns for law and order. The imperative need was to develop a sense of fear of authority in the entire population, and it was achieved through this system of the ruler's police. The police were to be shaped as an instrument of the Raj, one where men were disciplined, armed and without hesitation would follow British officers' orders' (Das and Verma,1998.).

The Act ipso facto continues to be operative. The only difference is that the 'British officer' is replaced by the 'Brown Sahib'. Little wonder then that between 2001 to 2010, 14,231 custodial deaths were recorded by the National Human Rights Commission (NHRC), i.e. on an average 4.33 persons died in police and judicial custody in India every day (Asian Centre For Human Rights, 2011). One can only hope that this example sufficiently graphically illustrates the point being made. I shall bolster it with examples specific to the health policy paradigm that has been pursued in India.

The recommendations of the Bhore Committee (its report was accepted by the government in 1946) constitute the most elaborate, liberal, and by far the most desirable of the schemes for the development of the health sector in the country that have yet been made. Even so, expressing its concerns regarding the population problem, the Committee said:

> A reduction in the rate of growth of population may be brought about by permitting the death rate in the community to rise. Our social instincts militate against this ...... One of the objectives universally accepted in all civilized countries is reduction of morbidity and mortality in the community. We have, therefore, to turn to other means of decreasing the rate of growth of population (GOI, 1946, Vol. II, pp. 483-4.).

It appears that but for the norms imposed by civilized countries, it might well have been recommended that 'the death rate (be allowed) to rise' as a means of controlling population growth. Their contempt for the people, nonetheless, is quite forthright. The Committee states further:

> A birth control campaign has certain inherent dangers ....Contraceptive practices are, therefore, more likely to be used by the more successful and intelligent sections of the community than by those who are improvident and mentally weak. It may also be mentioned that a certain number of defects, and diseases are known to be inheritable ... The *classes* (emphasis mine) which possess many of these undesirable characteristics are known to be generally *improvident and prolific* (emphasis mine). A continued high birth rate among these classes, if accompanied by a marked fall in the rate of growth of the more energetic, intelligent and ambitious sections of the population, which make much the largest contribution to the prosperity of the country, may be fraught with serious consequences to national welfare (GOI, 1946: Vol. II, p. 487).

There need be no confusion as to which class is being decried: precisely that which depends most on the services of public sector health care. There is a continuum, between 1946 and today, in the contempt that the rulers reserve for the commonest of common Indians. In 2009 the then Minister for Health and Family Welfare at the Centre commented:

> If there is electricity in every village, then people will watch TV till late at night and then fall asleep. They won't get a chance to produce children ... When there is no electricity there is nothing else to do but produce babies (Blackely, 2009.).

Class Character of the Ruling Elite and the Development of Health Services in India

Unlike the bourgeois democracies of the West, the democratic form of government in India did not evolve through a thorough going struggle encompassing the commonest of common Indians in a struggle for liberation. The bourgeois democratic 'format' of polity was imposed in India by the colonial rulers from above and adopted as such by the native '*Macaulayan*' élite. Therefore, while the better off among different sections of the society are co-opted in the ruling structure, the vast base of society has little space to democratically demand reforms and to assert themselves except within the limits defined by and the ways prescribed by the ruling classes.

True to their comprador class character, the rulers in India developed the health care system in the image of those prevalent in the developed capitalist countries rather than one that was sensitive to local needs and relied on the resources available in India.

India and China set out to meet their 'tryst with destiny' as modern states almost at the same time, with China actually two years behind (1949) India (1947). Both were ancient civilizations and repositories of some of the most ancient indigenous systems of medicine rooted in popular culture and enjoying widespread credibility among the people. The size of their populations, poverty, very low levels of development, widespread hunger and disease were other features common to both. Even so, the trajectories that the development of the health systems took in either country were remarkably divergent.

China relied on a mix of modern medical knowledge and the indigenous knowledge systems to turn around the health of its predominantly rural masses, and the agents of this change were not 'medical doctors' imbued with the technical finesse and the rigour of modern medicine, but millions of 'barefoot doctors' mobilized from among the impoverished, often illiterate peasant men and women. They were selected by their communities on the basis of their willingness to serve their communities; educated and trained using the resources the communities could afford with the active support of the state. The indigenous medical knowledge systems were integrated on an equal footing with modern medicine at all levels of health care: primary, secondary, and tertiary; and the science underlying the traditional systems was developed and made explicit. Many of the barefoot doctors were supported by the state to go on and become fully-fledged medical doctors and then return to serve their communities (Sidel and Sidel, 1973; 1982). Most importantly, this development was purely home grown, placing reliance almost exclusively on indigenous resources.

India's trajectory provides a study in contrast. The Bhore Committee, which otherwise made some laudable recommendations (many of which flowed from the recommendations made by the Dawson Committee and the Beveridge Committee reports produced in the UK in 1920 and 1942 respectively, for the development of health services in India, relied on the 'production of only one and that most highly trained type of doctor, which we have termed the "basic" doctor' (graduate of modern medicine) (GOI, 1946, Vol. II, p. 340). As opposed to this, the committee on National Health of the National Planning Committee of the Indian National Congress proposed:

> If medical advice and treatment to the mass of the people is to be provided on the necessary scale free of charge, the National Plan will have to bring the indigenous Vaidya, Hakim, or Dai into line with more elaborately or pretentiously trained physician or surgeon, gynecologist or obstetrician (Sokhey Committee, 1948).

That the latter were privileged over the former had its consequences, for after all which class could afford the latter. The Mudaliar Committee was of the opinion that:

> integration of Modern Medicine and Ayurveda is eminently desirable and all steps towards achieving that end should be promoted. Such integration should result in the development of a system of medical knowledge and practice based on all the best that is available in Modern Medicine and in Ayurveda. (Mudaliar Committee, 1959, p. 457.)

That such statements were intended merely for public consumption is evident from the assertion that:

> Participation in international health activities requires that the national health service in India should be based on modern medicine; the core of India's health service must continue to consist of persons adequately trained in Modern Medicine (Mudaliar Committee, 1959, p. 458).

The policy proactively sought to make medical education the exclusive preserve of the affluent. The Mudaliar Committee that followed the Bhore Committee endorsed the 'opinion of the conference of principles of Medical Colleges that English should continue to be the medium of instruction in the medical colleges' (Mudaliar Committee, 1959, p. 327). A further reflection of the mindset of the policy-planners is evident from the following comment in the Mudaliar Committee Report: reservation for

Scheduled Castes and backward communities, which is incumbent under the Constitution, have all tended to limit the number of well-qualified students being admitted to colleges' (Mudaliar Committee, 1959, p. 317).

Neither in 1960, when the Mudaliar Committee came out with its report, nor even today do the vast multitudes of the working classes in India endowed with proficiency in the English language, and indeed the worst off sections among are from the scheduled castes and the scheduled tribes. Therefore it is only the English speaking, urban based, rich upper class/upper caste students who can aspire for commanding positions in the health services/health policy system in India; or for that matter, in any other field of governance or white collar professions.

This automatically divides the population in two distinct sections: a miniscule minority of the well-endowed, urbane, civilized, intelligent, capable, and meritorious herd of technocrats, bureaucrats, the judiciary, captains of industry, officers of the armed forces, doctors, engineers, academics, etc. upon whom falls the task of caring for, tending to, educating, and developing the vast multitudes of the labouring poor who are deemed to be capable of little other than sell their labour. Much less than harness the energy and the potential of the poor to take their destiny into their own hands, such an institutionalized demarcation of the people places the downtrodden in perpetual positions of dependency. The 'White Man's Burden' thus into the 'Brown Sahib's Burden'.

Élitism is not just a matter of social status or the class to which one belongs, but also how one conceptualizes the problems and their solutions. For the élite who came to occupy dominating positions in India's health systems hierarchy, setting up large tertiary care hospitals and medical colleges with sophisticated machinery/technology was a far greater priority than setting up primary health care centres and sub-centres in rural areas; they had greater faith in technology-driven vertical disease control programmes, often imposed by international donor agencies, as an instrument of eliminating diseases rather than general health systems strengthening down to the village level as the strategic choice in overcoming morbidity and mortality (Banerji, 1985). Banerji writes that the rulers quoted the recommendations of the

Bhore Committee, often out of context, to draw legitimacy for their own plans to:

> establish a very large number of medical colleges with sophisticated teaching hospitals in urban areas. They also invoked the Bhore Committee to justify setting up an even more sophisticated All India Institute of Medical Sciences in New Delhi on the model of the Johns Hopkins Medical Centre of USA (quoting Mudaliar Committee Report, Vol. I, p. 191). A number of other postgraduate centres for medical education were also set up in due course. It however, took them over seven years even to start opening primary health centres to provide integrated curative and preventive services to rural populations of the country. These primary health centres were a very far cry from what was suggested by the Bhore Committee. (Banerji, 1977a)

There is sometimes a tendency to get carried away by 'socialist' notions and phrase-mongering regarding the leading role of the state in health care that were sought to be attached to these policies. With the benefit of hindsight one can say that the great power rivalry of the bipolar world afforded our rulers the luxury of appropriating notions of welfarism unto themselves even as they persistently pursued policies to favour big capital and the semi-feudal forces in India. The relative shifts between the Left and Right in terms of policies were guided more by the desire to extract concessions from one or the other superpower. However, the demise of the Soviet Union has revealed the true nature of our ruling élite, especially with the attendant ascendency of the neoliberalism as the dominant economic and social policy since the early 1990s.

Élitist Medical Education

Banerji mentions two diametrically opposite social objectives of medical education, one, 'to ensure that (the) educational system prepares physicians who are specially moulded to serve the requirements of the country'; secondly, 'to train professional physicians who are well-versed with the knowledge of modern medicine in its most sophisticated forms and who are trained mostly to provide services to those who can afford to pay for such services' (Banerji, 1977b).

Tables 10 and 11 help us gauge which of the two social objectives has been met by the medical education system in India.

With concerted efforts to bring about 'structural corrections' in the rural health care system in India through NRHM the

Table 10: Availability of Allopathic Doctors in the Rural Health care Set Up in India

Year	*2005***	*2007*	*2008*	*2010*	*2011*
Rural population	78,14,88,000*	79,99,05,000*	80,88,43,000*	82,61,73,000*	83,30,87,662
Total no. of government doctors in the rural health sector.(a)	23,858	27,725	28,654	42,584	45,062
Doctors/1000 of rural population	0.03	0.03	0.04	0.05	0.05
Total no. of government allopathic doctors (b)	67,576	76,542	84,852	85,254	97,648
Total no. of allopathic doctors registered with IMC/SMCs in India. (c)	6,60,801	7,31,439	7,61,429	8,46,172	9,21,877
Total no. of allopathic doctors in urban areas (c – a)	6,36,943	7,03,714	7,32,775	8,03,588	8,76,815
Ratio of the rural to urban allopathic doctors (c – a)/a	1:26.7	1:25.4	1:25.6	1:18.9	1:19.5

Source: *Figures for rural population for the respective years have been calculated from tables projected total population by sex in India (as on March 1, 2001 to 2026) and projected urban population by sex in India (as on March 1, 2001 to 2026) available from indiastat.com.

**Figures for 2005 have been taken from the comparative tables available in the *Bulletin of Rural Health Services* (RHS), *2011*. Figures for the respective years have been taken from the *RHS Bulletin* for the respective year.

Note: It needs be noted that the availability of doctors in the rural health services is the availability as on record. However, there are large variations in the actual availability of doctors in the rural health institutions due to problems like absenteeism, unequal posting of doctors at different institutions.

To calculate the total number of allopathic doctors (excluding dental surgeons) in urban areas we have presumed that government doctors posted in rural areas are the only allopathic doctors in rural areas, which is largely true with some variations. As regards the availability of allopathic doctors in urban areas, the figures are only approximations because we have presumed that all the doctors registered with the medical councils and are not serving in the rural health services to be working in urban areas, whereas in actuality many of them migrate overseas.

Table 11: Top 5 Countries for International Medical Graduates (IMG) Physicians Working in the US

Country	*Total IMG Physicians*	*% of Total IMG Population*
India	51,447	20.7
Philippines	20,601	8.3
Mexico	13,834	5.6
Pakistan	12,111	4.9
Dominican Republic	7,979	3.2

Total number of physicians in the US: 941,304Total number of IMG physicians-2,43,457 (from 127 countries)% IMG physicians in the US-26.0 %
Source: Tables 1 and 2 in AMA, 2010

Doctors per 1,000 population ratio in India has barely risen from 0.03 to 0.05. The total number of doctors available to serve the over 833 m. rural population in India in 2011 was a measly 45,062, while in 2007 this figure was only 27,725. It is sobering to note that in 2007 the number of Indian medical graduates working in the US alone was over 50,000 when the population of the US was just over 300 million.

AIIMS, the medical institute modelled along the lines of Johns Hopkins Medical Institute to train the model modern doctors of India, has indeed led from the front in bolstering the trend of migration of Indian doctors to greener pastures in the West. From 1989 to 2000 nearly 54 per cent of the medical graduates from the Institute migrated out of India. From amongst these graduates too, those from the better-off social backgrounds (the general category graduates were twice as likely to migrate, than those from the reserved categories) and those who performed better academically had a 35 per cent higher chance of migrating than those performing less well (Kaushik et al., 2008).

Of the remaining graduate doctors in India, nearly 74 per cent live in urban areas serving a mere 28 per cent of the population (Yadav et al., 2009), assuming that the urban poor have the wherewithal to access their services. The élite capture of medical education has meant that doctors being produced in India are largely from the privileged sections of the larger cities. The current form of medical education inculcates in them an a passion for technology-driven costly curative care in the increasingly corporatized health care of the cities in India or Western shores. The somewhat drab illnesses of the rural folk that have their origins principally in poverty and malnutrition naturally fail to attract attention.

The careerist and commercial motivations inherent in such an education naturally undermine the more holistic concerns such as the impact of poverty, caste, class, gender, and ethnic discrimination on health. This situation can only be exacerbated by the increasing commercialization of higher education that has already made it almost the exclusive preserve of the rich. There have been murmurs about 'reorienting' medical education and improving the clinical skills of medical graduates to address the health needs of the poor, but Thus far these promises have proved illusionary.

Rural-Urban Dichotomy in Health Services

It is in the nature of the systems based on exploitation that the backyards of exploitation are maintained to preserve the privileges of the few. The government's greatest concern is to first satisfy the needs of the urban élite. It is little wonder then that while the more affluent sections of rural society have gained upward mobility and have succeeded in coming closer to affording the amenities of the cities, including expensive curative facilities, but in the main the colonial paradigm of the rural-urban dichotomy in the provision of health service remains unchanged to this day.

CEHAT (Centre for Enquiry into Health and Allied Themes) undertook an exercise to disaggregate the health budget allocated to rural and urban areas from the finance accounts of five states from different parts of India for 2002-3. The results are shown in Table 12.

Table 12: Rural Urban Inequities in Public Health Expenditure of Selected States for the Year 2002-03

State/ Type of Expenditure		*Medical Care**	*Public Health*	*Family# Welfare*	*MCH*	*Capital***	*Total*	*Rural / Urban Population*
Maharashtra	Rural	5.71%	60%	49.97%	60%	0.78%	32.51%	66.57%
	Urban	94.29%	40%	50.03%	40%	99.2%	67.49%	42.43%
Mizoram	Rural	51.9%	51%	63.87%	51%	100%	55.68%	50.47%
	Urban	48.1%	49%	36.13%	49%	0.00%	44.32%	49.53%
Orissa	Rural	46.89%	80%	90.20%	80%	53.4%	58.89%	85.01%
	Urban	53.11%	20%	09.80%	20%	46.5%	41.11%	14.99%
Punjab	Rural	42.47%	66%	65.46%	0	0.00	45.00%	66.08%
	Urban	57.53%	34%	34.54%	0	100%	54.60%	33.92%
Tamil Nadu	Rural	18.96	54%	73.07%	54%	75.0%	35.01%	55.96%
	Urban	81.04	44%	26.49%	44%	24.7%	64.66%	44.04%
Madhya Pradesh	Rural	39.47	73%	72.80%	73%	90.6%	50.03%	73.54%
	Urban	60.53	27%	27.17%	27%	9.34%	49.96%	26.46%

Source: CEHAT, 2006. * Includes health services both allopathy and other system of medicines; minor head includes ESIS, Medical education dep., drug manufacture; # excluding MCH Programme; ** Includes capital expenditure on medical expenses, public health, and family welfare. The proportions of rural and urban population are taken from CBHI, 2005.

Note: Demarcation for the rural and urban health budget was effected from Finance Accounts 2002-3 for the respective states. For about two-thirds of the expenditure there is a clear rural-urban indication in the budget; for the rest, CEHAT used their functional knowledge of programme implementation to allocate proportions to rural and urban areas.

In the rural-urban distribution of the health budget it is noteworthy that with the exception of Mizoram, in no other state is the rural health budget allocated in proportion to the size of the rural population which is by far greater than the urban population. Secondly, it may be noted that the rural health budget largely comprises family welfare budgets, while for curative care the budget is heavily loaded in favour of the urban areas. It is our villages that are the hotbeds of poverty, caste discrimination, illiteracy, malnutrition, and disease. Apparently, our planners are concerned about the proliferation of this population, and therefore the need for increased allocation for family planning; whatever may become of the slogan, 'development is the most powerful contraceptive. Even if we were to disregard concerns for the functionality of rural beds, Table 13 further shows the preponderance of curative facilities in the urban areas, meaning thereby that rural-urban dichotomy is intertwined with what may be termed the curative-preventive dichotomy.

Table 13: Number of Government Hospital Beds in Rural and Urban Areas

State	*Rural Hospital Beds (govt.)*	*Urban Hospital Beds (govt.)*	*Total Beds (govt.)*	*Proportion of Rural and Urban Beds*
Bihar	1830	16686	18516	10:90
Chhattisgarh	3270	6158	9428	35:65
Jharkhand	N.A.	N.A.	N.A.	N.A.
Madhya Pradesh	10040	18493	28533	35:65
Odisha	7099	8715	15814	45:55
Rajasthan	13754	12236	25990	53:47
Uttar Pradesh	15450	40934	56384	27:73
Uttarakhand	3746	4219	7965	47:53
EAG states	55189	107477	162630	34:66
Non-EAG states	114673	511187	622310	18:82
All India	169862	618664	784940	20.5:79.5

Source: GOI, 2011.

Curative-Preventive Dichotomy in the Health Services

Beginning with Chadwick's sanitary reforms in the UK, the history of modern medicine is replete with evidence of how preventive measures have played a defining role in man's continuing struggle against disease, resulting in the elimination of many diseases as public health problem in the industrialized West. Much later, countries like China and Cuba showed the way to improving the health of entire populations by prioritizing disease prevention through comprehensive public health measures, and at a cost that is a fraction of spending otherwise incurred on cost-intensive technological interventions.

In India we seem to have learnt the lessons the other way round and medical technologies have become a substitute for taking action on more basic issues such as water, sanitation, and nutrition. For example, the massive 'Pulse Polio Programme' has been pushing unprecedented doses of polio vaccine, totally disregarding its impact on the epidemiology of the disease, while it having nothing to offer in terms of intervention in the principle mode of transmission of polio, i.e. faeco-oral transmission through contaminated water supply (Sathyamala, 2005; JSA, 2007). Tackling the latter would have benefits for a host of other public health problems such as diarrheal diseases, typhoid, and malnutrition. Similarly, the Revised National Tuberculosis Control Programme (RNTCP) has placed its bet only on providing DOTS (directly observed therapy short course) while leaving untouched the conditions that give rise to tuberculosis. The result has naturally been rising mortality due to TB (Dasgupta, 2012) and an increasing morbidity due to multi-drug resistant tuberculosis (Maurya et al., 2013). Undermining disease prevention only leaves us with the task of tackling a greater burden of morbidity and mortality at later stages and thereby placing the curative facilities under severe strain.

Table 14, based on figures in Table 3.7, National Health Accounts of India, 2004-5 provides the health expenditure by different ICHA (International Classification of Health Accounts) functions. Of the total health budget, the preventive functions command barely 20.78 per cent of the budget while curative services corner close to 50 per cent. The relatively higher proportion of preventive health care spending of the central government is because all the National Disease Control Programmes are funded by the Centre.

Table 14: Health Expenditure by ICHA Functions, National Health Accounts, 2004-05

	Health care Function	*Proportion of Budget Spent by*		
		*Center**	*State*	*Total*
HC.1	Curative care	22.16%	46.92%	42.67%
HC. 2 & 3	Rehabilitative and long-term nursing care	1.02%	0.13%	0.28%
HC.4	Ancillary services related to medical care	1.46%	2.50%	2.33%
HC.5	Medical goods dispensed to out-patients	2.01%	0.69%	0.92%
Sub-total	**Curative Health care Services**	**26.65%**	**50.24**	**46.2**
HC.6	Prevention and Public Health Services			

	RCH and Family Welfare	24.23%	9.55%	12.07%
	Control of Communicable Diseases	14.64%	5.20%	6.82%
	Control of Non-Communicable Diseases	01.63%	0.76%	0.91%
	Other Public Health Activities	1.24%	0.93%	20.78%
Sub-total	**Preventive Health care Services**	**41.74%**	**16.44%**	**20.78%**
HC.7	Health Administration and Insurance; Health and Related Functions (Medical Education and Training of Health Personnel, Research and Development, Capital Formation, Food Adulteration Control); Functions from Other Sources; Functions Not Specified.	31.61%	33.21%	31.86%
	Nutrition Programme	-	0.10%	0.08%
Sub-total	Health Functions Other Than Curative & Preventive	31.61%	33.31	31.94
	Total	**100**	**100**	**100**

Source: GOI, 2004-05.

Note: * is related to Ministry of Health and Family Welfare only.

1. Services of curative care include expenditure on teaching hospitals, specialty hospitals, ESI dispensaries, homeopathic hospitals, and dispensaries, ayurvedic hospitals and dispensaries, primary health centres, community health centres and expenditure on dental care, etc.
2. Rehabilitative care includes expenditure on rehabilitative centres for TB and leprosy patients, institute for the rehabilitation of the physically handicapped, drug de-addiction programmes, etc.
3. Ancillary services relating to medical care includes expenditure on blood banks, blood transfusion council, regional diagnostic centres, ambulance-related expenditure, medical store depot, etc.
4. RCH and family welfare covers expenditure on RCH and family welfare programmes.

The nutrition programme is included in Health and Related Functions but has been separately mentioned here on purpose. It would hardly be an exaggeration to say that 'Food is the basic medicine of public health' and yet at a conceptual and programmatic level the health planners seem to have completely divorced themselves from this. It is true that there are supplementary nutrition programmes run by other departments of the government, but should that be a reason for the health policy establishment to have almost given up on such a fundamental aspect that impacts on the health of the people as nothing else does, only to focus on narrow techno-centric approaches to alleviate the health problems of the people? After all, what is the worth of complete immunization to a malnourished child?

Market Led Growth of Health care in India

Internationally and from India there is a large body of literature (Hong, 2000; Gandy, M., 2005; Baru et al., 2010; Duggal, 1998; JSA, 2006; Bhide and Shand, 2000; Marriot, 2009) that attests to the devastating effects of market-led growth of health care. The biggest blow that globalization has dealt to health care systems is that it has uprooted health care from its moorings in 'social justice' and 'service' to humanity and legitimized it as a source of extracting profits. As already mentioned above, this paradigm shift governs not only the private sector, but has extended to the public sector health care in the form of commercialization of its components/ services. Paradoxically, the public sector has proved to be a supporting pillar for private health care in India. Public sector medical colleges contributed hugely to the growth of the private sector with 80 per cent of the doctors graduating from these colleges either joining the private sector or migrating overseas (Jan Swasthya Abhiyan, 2006b, p. 24).

Even though private health care always constituted a larger part of the health care system in India, with globalization, large corporate houses entered the health care provisioning and have increasingly influenced health policies and set standards of care that are far removed from the real-life conditions of ordinary Indians. The private sector constitutes eighty per cent of the health sector in India (Gangoli, 2005). Corporate health care is pushing high end technologies in both diagnostics and treatment irrespective of their desirability for the profile of public health problems in India. Additionally, promoting unjustifiably high end technologies is a drag on precious public resources for health either in the form of direct or indirect tax concessions on their import and operation and through public-private partnerships doled out to the private sector.

Now there is talk of the government turning itself into net purchaser of curative health care from the private sector while restricting itself to providing a small package of preventive services.

This has been euphemistically termed as 'managed care' (Dhar Aarti, 2012). The imposition and successive escalation of 'user charges' levied for the services of publically financed health institutions is another feature of neoliberal economic policies that is the bane of the poor (Bajpai and Saraya, 2010).

With corporate health-care becoming the 'prima donna' of the health-care industry in India, this has consequences for the motivation of public sector health workers in dedicating themselves to the more holistic motives of public health-care. The motivation of workers critically impacts the performance of the health sector as efficiency, equity, and service quality are all are directly transacted by the willingness of the workers to dedicate themselves to their tasks (Franco, 2002). Apart from individual level determinants, worker motivation is determined by 'organizational (work context) level, and determinants stemming from interactions with the broader societal culture' (Franco, 2002).

The 'broader societal culture' of health care today is being tempered by the commercialized ethos of private health care. For example, while the health care system allows for (implicitly or explicitly) a number of extraneous incentives, varying from systems of commissions from private diagnostic labs to outright bribes to doctors by drug and medical equipment manufacturers, not for their work to further patient care, but because of the position they occupy in the medical system, similar opportunities are not available to the other categories of hospital staff, who may then be tempted to resort to more crude and direct extraction of money from patients.

In either case, personal aggrandizement becomes the desired social objective and any improvement in the societal wellbeing becomes contingent upon the fulfilment of the former. These are not inadvertent outcomes but the result of the policies that have been pursued over the years. Developing markets in health-care has become the conscious objective of the economic and health policy of the state. Today the price for which the private sector plucks top notch consultants from public hospitals is considered a measure of the doctor's professional capabilities. The government on its part feigns helplessness notwithstanding the fact that it spent a considerable sum of people's money in first training these consultants and then affording them the facilities of public hospitals to hone their clinical skills. The private sector gobbles up the talent at virtually no cost to itself.

Another insult to injury that has been added during the implementation of the neoliberal economic policies since the beginning of the 1990s has been the large-scale hiring of contractual staff at all levels for work profiles that are perennial in nature. The contract paramedical and medical staff feels exploited even as they do more work than the regular health workers for lower remuneration and facilities. Such medical and paramedical health workers hardly visualize their future with the public hospital or public health system. For them such an engagement is a stop-gap measure which they must use for maximizing personal welfare rather than the welfare of their patients.

In all these years there has not been a single study to show that hiring staff on a contractual basis has helped in increasing the patient care or efficiency of hospitals yet the myth keeps getting reinforced that contractual staff can be made to work better than the regular staff because it suits the convenience of the government and the administrators.

The private medical sector has proved to be the proverbial 'camel' that has pushed the Arab (the public medical sector') out of the tent.

Deficiency of Political Will

As goes the adage, 'where there is a will, there is a way', equally true is our contention that 'where there is no will, there are alibis and subterfuge, albeit in the form of elaborate schemes'. No government in India since the 1947 transfer of power has failed to express its solidarity with the Indian masses in terms of alleviating their suffering. On the face of it, they still remain committed to increase welfare spending cutting across the political spectrum. However, the failure to achieve up to now even the goals and targets laid out for the first ten year period after independence in the Bhore Committee Report is a significant pointer.

In 1977, India's ruling classes committed themselves to the Alma Ata Declaration on achieving 'Health care For All by the year 2000' through the strategy of Primary Health Care. No sooner than this commitment was made, our ruling élites jumped on to the bandwagon of Selective Primary Health Care that was sponsored by the American foundations and multinational vaccine corporations. The year 2000 came and went, but the goals of neither Primary Health Care nor its 'selective' variant were achieved.

Come 2002, the then Bharatiya Janata Party led National Democratic Alliance came up with the National Health Policy and soon thereafter was the National Common Minimum Programme of the first United Progressive Alliance government eminently supported by the parliamentary left. Both promised to increase the health spending to a level of 2 to 3 per cent of the GDP by 2010 (Chaudhary, 2006). A huge programme for the renewal of rural health care in India was launched in the form of the National Rural Health Mission (NRHM) in 2005. Having completed its first phase of seven years in 2012 without having been able to achieve even one of the goals set before it, the NRHM is now into its second phase. Even so, the pious objective of taking the public health expenditure in the country to 2 to 3 per cent of the GDP continues to elude India.

At the time of rolling out the process of preparing their Programme Implementation Plans (PIP) for the implementation of the NRHM during the financial year 2013-14, the states were instructed that they could increase their expenditure under NRHM up to 30 per cent over the baseline of 2012-13 but in the meanwhile the economic slowdown hit back and by the time of actual allocation of central assistance to the various states, the officials of the Ministry of Health and Family Welfare bluntly told the states that no increase in allocation would be possible (I was privy to these developments while working as a consultant with the National Health Systems Resource Centre, Government of India).

Apart from signifying the size of the resource package, the health budget is important inasmuch as this is the single most important measure of the political commitment of the rulers to improve the health of the people. The government backing off from offering even a very modest increase in the budget for rural health-care at the first whiff of an economic slowdown, even as it continues to offer tax exemptions to the wealthiest to the tune of lakhs of crores of rupees, shows the shakiness of their political commitment to the welfare of the people.

As to the possibility of doing things differently, I present the comparison between Cuba and India to underscore what political commitment to health care means. It is well known that Cuba went through a sudden and catastrophic economic crisis in the early 1990s due to the collapse of the Soviet Union and along with it the collapse of the preferential trade and economic aid Cuba received from the Soviets. The Cuban economy contracted suddenly and rapidly. These are the kind of trying circumstances that test the commitment of governments to ensure human well-being as reflected by the resources committed for this. Generally speaking, the experience is that in times of economic crisis, expenditure on welfare (health, education, and food) is the first to come under the knife, precisely at a time when the people, especially the poor, need additional protection.

Beginning in the 1990s, India also faced an onerous economic crisis which queered the pitch for neoliberal economic reforms. Tables 15 and 16 present the response of the governments of Cuba and India towards ensuring human welfare under such trying circumstances. After the economic crisis, the total government expenditure declined continually till 1998 compared to the base year of 1989, except for a marginal increase in 1991 and 1992. There was also an absolute decline in expenditure on social services, almost continually till 1994, after which the absolute budgetary allocation for social services began increasing once more even though the total budget of the government was still contracting compared to that of the base year. As a proportion of total government expenditure, however, expenditure on social services began recovering from 1992 itself. The budget on social services varied between 16.5 to nearly 20 per cent. Cuba severely compromised on its defence budget which was reduced from 9.04 per cent of the total government expenditure in 1989 to 4.1 per cent in 1998. This is exceptional given the geopolitical situation of Cuba, especially at a time when it was most vulnerable to US hostility.

Table 15: Cuba's Total Government Expenditure and Expenditure on Social Services (including health) and Defence During the Special Period (in Millions of Current Pesos)

Year	*Total Government Expenditure*	*Expenditure on Defence/Internal Order*	*Expenditure on Social Services (Education & Health)*
1989	14041	1269 (9.04%)	2576 (18.35%)
1990	13852	1120 (8.1%)	2492 (18.00%)
1991	15436	925 (6.0%)	2548 (16.50%)
1992	14312	746 (5.2%)	2395 (16.70%)
1993	12564	615 (4.9%)	2123 (16.90%)
1994	10035	461 (4.6%)	1696 (16.90%)
1995	8866	392 (4.42%)	1584 (17.90%)
1996	8326	323 (3.9%)	1697 (20.4%)
1997	8368	421 (5.03%)	1797 (21.50%)
1998	8344	343 (4.1%)	1823 (21.80%)

Source: Based on data given in Table 5, Dunning, 2001.

With respect to India the situation is almost the reverse. Our defense expenditure has consistent varied between 14 to 15.5 per cent during the 1990s, whereas expenditure on social services hovered between 3 to 5 per cent.

Table 16: India's Total Government Expenditure and Expenditure on Social Services (including Health) and Defence During the Economic Crisis of Early 1990s (in Billion Current Rupees)

Year	*Total Government Expenditure*	*Defence Expenditure*	*Social Services Expenditure*
1989-90	929.08	144.16 (15.5%)	30.61 (3.3%)
1990-1	1052.98	154.26 (14.6%)	32.74 (3.1%)
1991-2	1114.14	163.47 (14.7%)	35.69 (3.2%)
1992-3	1226.18	175.82 (14.3%)	40.09 (3.3%)
1993-4	1418.53	218.45 (15.4%)	48.30 (3.4%)
1994-5	1607.39	232.45 (14.5%)	58.73 (3.7%)
1995-6	1782.75	268.56 (15.1%)	76.55 (4.3%)
1996-7	2010.07	295.05 (14.7%)	96.72 (4.8%)
1997-8	2320.53	352.78 (15.2%)	118.45 (5.1%)
1998-9	2793.4	398.97 (14.3%)	146.56 (5.2%)

Source: Based on figures taken from Tables 103 and 104, RBI, 2012-13

Figure 4 shows that India's public expenditure on health reached its nadir in 2004 when it accounted for barely 21 per cent of the total health expenditure. Between 2004 and 2011, this proportion increased from 21 per cent to 31 per cent, which can be directly attributed to the NRHM. However, the overall impact of this increase can be judged from the fact that it has made little difference to the overall expenditure on health in India. Indeed, there is a slight negative slope between 2004 and 2011 in the graph in this context. What is particularly noteworthy is that the phenomenally high economic growth-rates prevalent during the 1990s and 2000s seem to have made negligible difference to the overall resources being committed to health. An increase of 10 per cent in public expenditure as a proportion of the total expenditure on health is too little too late, and even this could well be set to suffer a rollback in the face of economic uncertainties that currently facing India.

Fig. 4: Variation in India's Health Expenditure with GDP Growth Rate

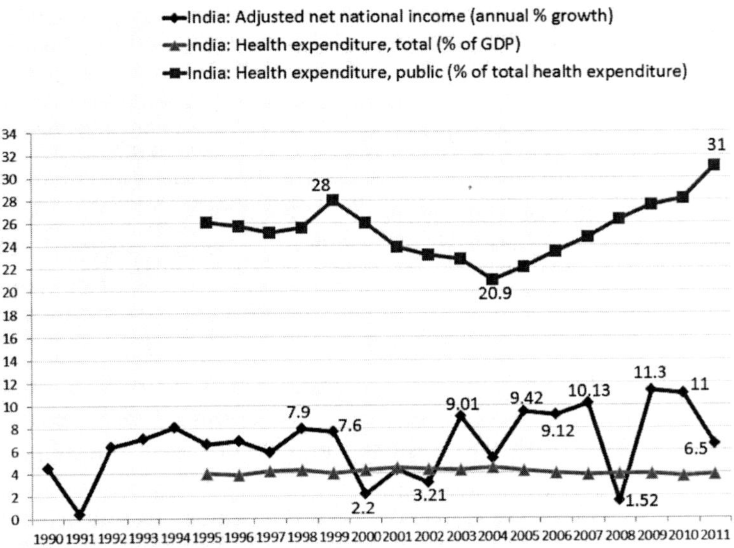

Source: All the figures have been obtained from Health Nutrition and Population Statistics in the World Bank databank. Available from http://databank.worldbank.org/data/views/variableselection/selectvariables.aspx?source=health-nutrition-and-population-statistics and accessed on August 15, 2013.

How Do We Overcome These Challenges?

Before we go on to discuss the possible solutions to the crisis under discussion, one has to be discerning about what is remediable and what is not under the social, political, and economic system currently prevalent in India. Tackling factors such as the class character of the ruling élite and their orientation towards development issues is a far more complex issue that can scarcely be remedied by some policy initiatives. The policy orientation of the ruling classes also depends upon larger global geopolitics. Bringing about a longer-lasting change in their character however entails a political process which is beyond the pale of our discussion here, except that an understanding of these issues enables us to make realistic assessments and policy choices that are feasible, besides aligning ourselves with the larger processes of political change. As a corollary, it also follows that even the most liberal policy regime that can be pursued in the given system will serve only as a partial solution of the crisis. However, even these partial solutions are worth pursuing insofar as they hold the promise of bringing some relief to the people from the present neoliberal policy regime.

With this caveat, we can say that the policy instruments to improve the functioning of public hospitals cannot but flow from an understanding of the consequences of the factors that constitute the crisis and their social and political origins. The solutions would essentially lie in instituting policies that would reverse these consequences.

The most fundamental premise underlining these solutions is that the provision of food, health care, water, sanitation, and education, the most important factors impacting on health outcomes ought to be ensured as a matter of right, free from profit motives. Also, only such measures can be acknowledged as solutions that are primarily responsive to the epidemiological needs of patients, rather than those that suit the exigencies of the health administrators.

It would be worthwhile to point out here the experience of the India's largest and the most reputed public health institution, the All India Institute of Medical Sciences (AIIMS).

Doctors at AIIMS have been complaining for a long time that

the huge daily rush of patients' in the Institute's outpatient department has not only worsened the standard of clinical care at the hospital, but barely leaves the faculty with time to concentrate on medical research and teaching. This is defeating the most important role that the Institute is supposed to perform, of setting up a model of patient care and medical teaching in India.

While one may disagree with the models they may have in mind, this is a perfectly legitimate concern of the faculty and administration at AIIMS. However, in response to this, various departments have arbitrarily decided to limit the number of patients registered daily in their outpatient departments. While this may have been expedient for institute administration to overcome its problem, the remedy has proved to be the quintessential double whammy for patients who come from the far corners of India to seek treatment at the AIIMS. It also seems unlikely that this solution will change things substantially. On the contrary, some senior doctors discovered (as personally related to me) that this 'solution' resulted in outpatient cards being sold at a high premium by some unscrupulous employees.

Worse still, developing models for excellence in patient care or for medical research in India does not seem to be an important motivation for such decisions. Most of the doctors have been passive in opposing the commercialization of services of such institutions, or in opposing attempts at privileging industry interest in their research. Doctors have been raising their economic demands but invariably fail to demand alternative strategies that are required to tackle the high patient load, or raise the issue of re-invigorating the peripheral health care institutions so that institutions like the AIIMS do not end up performing the functions of general hospitals. In fact, the height of cynicism on these issues can be judged from a comment made by a senior ex-faculty member of the institute in a conversation with me. While lamenting the falling standards of patient care due to the huge patient load, he went so far as to suggest: 'let the patients die (due to limited registration of patients), but the Institute must not let its standards be diluted.' It is not my claim that this view is shared by all the doctors at the AIIMS, but it certainly shows how retrogressive such a sentiment is.

Suggestions for Re-invigorating Peripheral Services and Improving the Services of Public Hospitals

For Reinvigorating Peripheral Services

- The task of making the primary and secondary level health institutions functional ought to be the utmost priority, such that people can access effective health care for common and easily treatable conditions at hospitals in proximity to their homes.
- Urgent steps need be taken to provide working and living conditions in the peripheral areas that will encourage doctors and other health personnel to be willing to opt for rural service. Family hostels should be built in the nearby urban centres to house the families of doctors and other medical personnel when they are posted in remote areas. The state should ensure the admission of their children to the best schools in the area and provide other such facilities. It may be noted that such steps are routinely taken in relation to defence personnel.
- All the vacancies for medical and paramedical posts should be promptly filled and the administrative procedures should facilitate speedier permanent appointments. There is little evidence to show that provision of ad hoc/contract appointments has led to a sustained availability of health personnel in rural areas.
- Consequent to fulfilment of the conditions, set out above, rural service should be made compulsory for health personnel of varying categories immediately after graduation. There should not be waivers of any kind to allow the personnel to avoid doing such service.
- Much greater reliance should be placed on the training of a large number of paramedical personnel or on reviving licentiate courses to fill the gap in the availability of primary level health care.
- The capacity of peripheral health services should be expanded to absorb the large number of health workers as full-time workers in the health services system. Private practice for any category of workers should not be permitted.

- Regular programmes should be organized requiring senior doctors from the secondary or tertiary level health facilities and medical colleges to mandatorily visit rural areas to help the peripheral health workers improve their knowledge and skills.
- Once these conditions are realized, certain administrative steps can be taken to ensure a proper referral system for the patients from the most peripheral to the tertiary level institutions.
- The local communities, peoples organizations, and representative bodies should be involved in 'the planning, organization, operation and control of primary health care, making fullest use of local, national, and other available resources' in the true spirit of primary health care, as enunciated in the Alma-Ata Declaration of 1977 (WHO, 1978). However, it needs to be stressed here that unless a fundamental reordering is brought about in the power relations of caste, class, gender, and community in rural society, the control and participation suggested here will only be exercised by the current dominant sections of rural society.
- Public hospitals associated with large institutes or medical colleges should be encouraged to further strengthen their outreach services.
- In order to ensure that things work as they ought to a system of accountability should be in place with the guiding principle that first responsibility has to be fixed on the most empowered functionary rather than the least empowered; and secondly, that no system of accountability can be enforced through policing oversight as the principal mechanism. In order to make people willing to be accountable, it is of utmost importance to provide a working environment that harnesses people's enthusiasm to work to the best of their respective capabilities.

It needs to be emphasized here that it is the ingrained logic of systems based on exploitative relations of production to believe that people work either in response to fear of authority or for individual material incentives. Such systems do not recognize the fundamental human need to engage in socially productive work.

Improving Services at Public Hospitals

- To reinvigorate the positive spirit of the Bhore Committee recommendations it needs to be stressed that national health organization ought to be a 'whole-time salaried service devoting itself to the development of the health of the people'. Therefore, the provision of allowing private practice by government doctors should be banned forthwith.
- For maximal utilization of the infrastructure of public hospitals, provision should be made for both morning and evening OPDs. The necessary staff, equipment, and space should be provisioned for running such clinics and diagnostic set-up. Evening OPDs should have the added advantage of obviating 'opportunity costs' for the poor who lose their daily wage to visit the hospital in the morning. It may be noted that if private hospitals and/or diagnostic centre can operate such facilities, why should it be difficult for a public hospital to do so?
- A number of modern technologies have become available over the years to improve the functioning of public hospitals. The guiding principle for their use should be that they should be used to maximize patient welfare, rather than to curtail patient services.

  Diagnostic equipment such as auto-analysers that are now available have replaced the manual diagnostic processes and can be deployed to undertake laboratory investigations round the clock without necessarily having to deploy larger manpower as was necessary with manual processes. This can be most useful to arrive at an early diagnosis of ailment and facilitate setting up of evening OPDs. Similarly, the use of information technology to improve hospital records; for example the laboratory or radiological investigations can be uploaded on a central portal so that they are readily available to those who have to use the results of the investigations. Such a measure can be very helpful in preventing harassment patients face while their reports are being traced, often ending up wasting days on this without actual movement in the treatment that they seek.

- Last but not least, all measures directed at commercializing the use of hospital services through imposition of user fees on patients should be abolished. These are highly inefficient in providing cross-subsidies to poor patients and have grave implications for equity and access to health care (Bajpai and Saraya, 2010).

The World Bank was the chief proponent of the imposition of user fees in public health services throughout the world. However, addressing the 66th World Health Assembly at Geneva on May 21, 2013 the World Bank President Jim Yong Kim said: 'Anyone who has provided health care to poor people knows that even tiny out-of-pocket charges can drastically reduce their use of needed services. This is both unjust and unnecessary' (Jim Yong Kim, 2013).

Reversing Market-Led Growth of Health care

Market-led growth of health care is part of the economic agenda of the ruling classes and is motivated by their 'class interests' which are in an antagonistic relationship with the 'class interests' of the working masses. Besides harnessing health care as a source of profit, the interest of the ruling classes is to provide exclusive services for the affluent sections of society while relegating public health services to a secondary status. The interest of the overwhelming mass of people, on the other hand, lies in the provisioning of universal health care as a 'societal good' irrespective of the individual's ability to pay.

If there is willingness to search for policy options based on the empirical examination of different policies that have been implemented in different parts of the world in different contexts, as also in India over the past two decades, there may perhaps be some scope of reasoning our way through to secure the interests of the common people. Unfortunately, as things stand today, such a possibility does not seem to exist.

The lack of political will on part of the government to act in the interest of the vast majority of poor people is linked to the class interests of the people it actually represents. In other words, the question is of class struggle which is part of a larger political process. Here I can only reiterate the need to choose sooner rather than later on whose side we are in this struggle.

As regards the government, it has made its intensions very clear by the fact that the Planning Commission rejected the High Level Expert Group (HLEG) *Report on Universal Health Coverage for India* which was instituted by the Commission itself.

The report, while being agreeable to private sector involvement in the health sector, had recommended 'expansion and augmentation of primary health care, strengthening of district hospitals, expansion and upgrading the skills of the health workforce, free provision of essential medicines, abolition of "user fees", establishment of effective regulatory structures and support for active community participation as high priorities requiring early action' (Reddy, 2012). Apart from the recommendation of contracting out services to the private sector wherever necessary, the HLEG recommended that 'every citizen should be entitled to assured free access to a package of essential health services, which will be periodically defined by an expert body, through a national health entitlement card (India Health Card). Public facilities for health care will have to be the main delivery system of UHC' (Reddy, 2012).

However, no sooner were these recommendations made by the HLEG, the system struck back. We have seen earlier in Chapter 3, how the World Bank, the Planning Commission and the government derailed possible rejuvenation of public health services system through the implementation of the HLEG report.

These developments regarding the HLEG recommendations, which in no way sought to establish 'socialism' in the sphere of health care delivery in the country, only point to the tenacity with which we need to pursue a pro-people health agenda in India.

Resolving the Question of Elitist Medical Education

As a measure of what is missing in our medical education today, I would like to quote from the Bhore Committee's Report:

> ... a social outlook should be developed in every health worker and that a spirit of emulation be cultivated throughout the rank and file of service....Understanding and sympathy, tact and patience are

> equally important for the proper handling of these persons and, in their absence, mere professional skill will fail to achieve satisfactory results. On the other hand the possession of these qualities will lift the efforts of the health worker to the plane of social service. (GOI, 1946, Vol. 2, p. 27)

'Dymystifying' medical education is an important task at hand. In order to make medical education the exclusive preserve of the élite there is a cultivated notion that medicine as a field of study is so complex that only those with exceptional intelligence and 'merit' can become worthy doctors. Above all, becoming a worthy doctor is a matter of having the aptitude to serve and that the real merit of a doctor does not lie as much in his/her being able to acquire medical knowledge, as much it lies in his/her ability to translate this knowledge into practice in highly challenging circumstances of our people and in the generation of new knowledge. These two later aspects have been totally sidelined in the manner of selection of medical students and their training.

As with other biological sciences, medical knowledge is more factual than logical or conceptual, which means that as far as acquiring medical knowledge is concerned one can do so by putting in a reasonable amount of hard work provided of course other impediments in accessing medical knowledge can be overcome. In my view there are four major impediments that need to be tackled forthwith:

- Dual system of education:

  The roots of the élite capture of the medical profession, and indeed other professional courses lies in the dual system of school education in the country: expensive English medium education for the élite and low quality government schools teaching in the vernacular medium. Education is not just about the medium of instruction but about inculcation of social, moral, and ethical values; it is about how one relates to and aspires to improve the society in which one lives. The top-notch English medium schools in the large urban centres have become a preserve of the rich who seek an exclusivist education for their children.

  So long as this class with exclusivist nurturing exists, they will seek and also manage almost exclusive access to top positions in all walks of life including the polity, the bureaucracy, the judiciary, and higher education. This is a class that is least desirous of sharing its privileges with the common citizenry and is by far the most potent force in the reproduction of the system as it stands today. Therefore the dual system of education must go.

- The present system of selection of medical graduates:
  The present system of medical entrance examination with its emphasis on memorizing more and more obscure facts and correctly recalling them while answering the multiple choice questions should be done away with. Over the years this system has spawned a whole industry of coaching institutes which provide this specialized training to crack the exams at prices that are invariably beyond the capacity of even many of the middle class families.
  Instead, a system of selection needs to be developed that will test the basic intelligence of the aspirants; their aptitude to serve the people, especially the underprivileged; their understanding of social issues impacting on the health of the people and other such factors. This could entail a multi-level selection process with each step being designed to sieve in the most deserving candidates.
  Towards this end we can learn from the historical examples that are available from post-1917 Soviet Union and pre-neoliberal reform China, but even the more contemporary examples like the 'National Training Programme for Comprehensive Community Physicians' (NTPCCP) in Venezuela (Cruz and Perea, 2008).
- De-commercialization of medical education:
  In order that men and women, and boys and girls from the subaltern sections of society can easily afford to receive a medical education it should be entirely free for all students with strict conditions built into the programme that the student will have to serve the underserved populations once they have completed their training. Such conditions should not be bartered for monetary or any other kind of fines.
  The upper age limit should be liberally relaxed to enable even older persons to receive medical education. For

candidates from working class or poor rural backgrounds the government should provide a maintenance allowance for the family so that the students can complete their education without having to worry about the needs of their families. Such measures have currently been undertaken in Venezuela as part of the NTPCCP.

Such reforms in medical education would automatically dis-incentivize it for those candidates who view medicine solely as a lucrative career option and help in changing the class base of the medical profession.

- Changing the medium of instruction from English to the locally spoken languages:

  In the Indian context, as perhaps might be true of many other developing countries, English is not just another language spoken by a certain section of people. It has come to represent a social class; is associated with certain social status, a cultural mindset, and, above all, is the language of governance in India. All this alienates an overwhelming majority of Indians who either do not have a knowledge of the language or a sufficient command of it from vast areas of governance, higher education, and élite professions where English is the transactional medium.

  An impression is created that our education, especially technical education, will lag behind international standards if the medium of instruction were not to be English. One need only point out here that barring the Anglo-Saxon world, English is not the currency of academic exchange in large parts of the world such as China, Japan, Russia, France, Germany, and the like, and can it be said that they lag behind international standards?

  We can devise some practical steps to make the transition, for example:

  A national project should be instituted to translate/write medical books into/in local languages while retaining the English technical terms with or without the corresponding term in the local language. For example, gall bladder can remain gall bladder for instruction in all languages or the word enzyme can be retained as such.

Till such time that an Indian language can be developed to act as a truly pan-Indian language, there will still be the need to impart a working knowledge of English, or communication skills in it, to all students to enable medical professionals across the country to engage in professional interaction.

While being discussed in the context of medical education, such measures need to be initiated in almost all the educational disciplines. In fact, one such beginning has been made in the state of Madhya Pradesh, and that too by a right wing political force such as the BJP. The President Pranab Mukherjee laid the foundation-stone of the Atal Bihari Vajpayee Hindi University at Mugalia Kot in the state on the June 7, 2013. The university has been established with the promise of offering courses in medicine and engineering, among others, in Hindi (Express News Service, 2013). It is to be seen however, how far this move goes, but it is a commendable beginning.

Apart from the measures discussed above, another important policy thrust has to be to bridge the gap between the medical and the paramedical branches of health care personnel. Policy measures should be devised to encourage the lower rungs of health care professionals, such as the nursing staff, ANMs, community health workers to graduate to the higher levels. Necessary changes should be made in the medical curricula/courses to facilitate this.

A word needs to be said here regarding the 'Rural Doctors' course that was being discussed some time ago. While being open to the desirability of such a course, I would caution that such a course should not end up as being a 'poor doctor' course for poor people and add another tier to the medical hierarchy. Instead, we need to consider devising a single uniform course at the undergraduate level that is much abridged and more focused on community level health care. The present MBBS course incorporates an excess of detailed information on many subjects that are really required only by a specialist in those subjects rather than a public health physician. Subjects such as forensic medicine can best be avoided at the undergraduate level.

These recommendations are only suggestive. I am certain that if a systematic approach is taken in this direction, far more constructive opinions can come forth.

Resolving the Curative-Preventive Dichotomy

The curative-preventive dichotomy in health is bound up with two things: the rural-urban dichotomy (preventive care for rural areas and costly curative care for urban areas), on the one hand, and on the other, the hierarchy between the curative and preventive branches of medicine. While the value of preventive medicine is not much appreciated by people in the absence of disease, seeking care becomes incumbent upon falling ill and therein lies the higher market value of clinical disciplines. To this extent, clinical care serves as a convenient avenue for profit generation. Therefore, the market-driven growth of health care has widened the gulf between the clinical and preventive branches, thereby increasing the overall cost of improving people's health. The following policy measures can be useful in bringing about a correction of this dichotomy:

- The overall development of public health care systems should minimize the profit motive in medicine and can be expected to privilege the application of preventive medical knowledge to reduce the overall cost of improving people's health.
- To strengthen curative care in rural areas by creating facilities that will encourage doctors and other paramedical personnel to accept postings in rural areas. The government cannot shy away from providing adequate boarding and lodging facilities for doctors besides taking care of family needs such as schooling for their children.

  An increasing number of training institutes should be located in rural areas for at least the lower categories of paramedical staff by upgrading the existing facilities.
- A necessary change needs to be brought about in the orientation of medical education as distinct from the efforts hitherto being made to reorient the medical curriculum.

> There is a need to include strong social science components in medical education to enable medical professionals to comprehend the complex social, economic, and political context in which medicine operates. Secondly, the clinicians should, as a matter of routine, be pulled out of their ivory towers to engage in preventive care/involved in strengthening preventive and promotive services.

Conclusion

In the context of the challenges facing public hospitals in India, it need to be remembered that the sorry state of affairs of public health-care is not for want of policies, managerial skills, or the most up-to-date technologies. The situation is what it is because it suits the interests of the dominant classes in society. To undo this situation requires much more than a bureaucratic or technocratic putsch. It demands popular mobilization of the widest possible sections of society, especially the working people, to support policy initiatives directed at demolishing the élite capture of health care and the medical profession in India.

From a hospital administrator's point of view, this account would indeed be very disappointing as there are no ready-made shortcuts on offer to improve the outcomes. Nonetheless, it is important to realize that health is a social phenomenon and a public hospital is a social institution which cannot be studied in isolation from the societal conditions within which it operates. The analysis presented here is in conformity with this reality. However, I am certain that there still are public hospitals that offer much to learn in terms of their internal functioning to improve the services of the rest.

Taken overall, the public health care system in India stands at the crossroads with little in the present system that is worth *emulating*. However, even as the adversities appear to be insurmountable, the solution lies in propagating and creating space for an alternative paradigm both in the realm of theory and practice. In order that theory gains in strength it must develop the language to articulate people's struggles for an alternative development paradigm.

REFERENCES

Asian Centre for Human Rights (2011): *Torture in India, 2011*, Asian Centre for Human Rights, November.

American Medical Association (AMA) (2010): 'International Medical Graduates in American Medicine: Contemporary Challenges and Opportunities', a position paper by the AMA-IMG Section Governing Council, January. Available from http://www.ama-assn.org/resources/doc/img/international-medical-graduates-in-american-medicine.pdf accessed on October 4, 2013.

Bhola, N., R. Kumari, T. Nidha (2008): 'Utilization of the Health care Delivery System in a District of North India,' *East African Journal of Public Health*, December, Vol. 5(3): 147-53.

Blackely, R. (2009): 'Ghulam Nabi Azad Says late Night TV Will Help Slow India's Birth Rate', *Sunday Times*, 13 July.

Banerji, D. (1985): *Health and Family Planning Services in India: An Epidemiological, Socio-cultural and Political Analysis and a Perspective* (New Delhi: Lok Paksh), pp. 23–6.

Banerji, D. (1977a): 'Evolution of Health Services in India', in *In Search of Diagnosis – Analysis of Present System of Health Care*, ed. Ashwin J. Patel, published by (Delhi: Voluntary Health Association of India for Medico Friend Circle), p. 15.

Banerji, D. (1977b): 'Objectives of Medical Education' in *In Search of Diagnosis: Analysis of Present System of Health Care*, ed. Ashwin J. Patel, (New Delhi: Medico Friend Circle).

Bhide, S. and Ric Shand (2000): 'Inequalities in Income Growth in India Before and After Reforms', *South Asia Economic Journal*, Vol. 1(1): 19-51.

Bajpai, V., and A. Saraya (2010): 'User Charges as a Feature of Health Policy in India: A Perspective', *National Medical Journal of India*, Vol. 23 (3): 163-70.

Baru, R., A. Acharya, S. Acharya et al. (2010): 'Inequities in Access to Health Services in India: Caste, Class and Region', *Economic and Political Weekly*, Vol. 45 (38): 49-58.

Chandra, N. (2012): 'Delhi Hospital Pays Hhigh Price for Excellence', *India Today*, June 10. Accessed from http://indiatoday.intoday.in/story/delhi-hospital-pays-high-price-for-excellence/1/200025.html on August 15, 2013.

Chaudhary, M. (2006): 'Public Spending on Health in Low-Income States and Central Transfers', Financing Human Development, Policy Brief, No. 1, September, National Institute of Public Finance and Policy.

Centre for Enquiry into Health and Allied Topics (CEHAT) (2006): 'Changing Health Budgets', Centre for Enquiry into Health and Allied Themes, Research Centre of Anusandhan Trust, May.

CBHI (2005): 'Table 1.1.3, National Health Profile, 2005' (New Delhi: Ministry of Health and Family Welfare, Government of India, Available from CBHI (Central Bureau of Health Intelligence) at http://cbhidghs.nic.in/CBHI%20Book/chapter1.pdf accessedon September 5, 2013.

Cruz, E.R.B. and R.S.S. Perera (2008): 'National Training Program for Comprehensive Community Physicians, Venezuela', *MEDICC Review*, Vol. 10 (4): 35-42.

Dhar, Aarti (2012): 'Activists Up in Arms Against New Proposal on Health Care', *The Hindu*, August 8, 2012.

Dunning, T. (2001): 'Structural Reform and Medical Commerce: The Political Economy of Cuban Health Care in the Special Period', Depart. of Political Science, University of California, Berkeley. Paper was prepared for delivery at the 2001 meeting of the Latin American Studies Association, Washington D.C., September 6-8, 2001. Available from lasa.international.pitt.edu/Lasa2001/DunningThad.pdf, accessed on August 31, 2013.

Das, D.K., and A. Verma (1998): 'The Armed Police in the British Colonial Tradition: The Indian Perspective', *Policing: An International Journal of Police Strategies & Management*, Vol. 21 (2): 354-67.

Dasgupta, R. (2012): 'Connecting the DOTS: Spectre of a Public Health Iatrogenesis?', *Indian Journal of Community Medicine*, Vol. 37 (1): 13-15.

Duggal, R. (1998): 'Health Care and New Economic Policies; The Further Consolidation of the Private Sector in India', Paper Presented at the National Seminar on the Rights to Development, University of Mumbai, December 10–11 (Mumbai: CEHAT), December.

Express News Service (2013): 'New MP Varsity to Teach Medicine, Engg in Hindi', *Indian Express*, June 7. Available from http://www.indianexpress.com/news/new-mp-varsity-to-teach-medicine-engg-in-hindi/1126170/accessed on September 6. 2013.

Franco, L.M., Sara Bennettb, Ruth Kanfer (2002): 'Health Sector Reform and Public Health Worker Motivation: A Conceptual Framework Resource', *Social Science and Medicine,* Vol. 54: 1255–6.

Ghosh, S. (2010): 'Catastrophic Payments and Impoverishment Due to Out-of-Pocket Health Spending: The Effects of Recent Health Sector Reforms in India', Asia Health Policy Programme working paper #15, Working paper series on Health and Demographic Change in the Asia-Pacific, Stanford University, Walter H. Shorenstein Asia-Pacific Research Centre Asia Health Policy Programme, July.

Government of India (1946): *Health Survey and Development Committee Report (Bhore Committee Report),* Vol. II (Delhi: Government of India Press).

Government of India (2013): *Rural Health Statistics 2012* (New Delhi: Ministry of Health and Family Welfare).

Government of India (2010): *District Level Household and Facility Survey 2007-08* (New Delhi: Ministry of Health and Family Welfare).

Government of India (2006): *Morbidity, Health care and the Condition of the Aged* (New Delhi: NSSO, Ministry of Statistics and Programme Implementation), March.

Government of India (2015): 'NSS 71st Round: Key Indicators of Social Consumption in India, Health', Ministry of Statistics and Programme Implementation, June.

Government of India (2004-5): *National Health Accounts 2004-05 (With Provisional Estimates from 2005–06 to 2008–09)* (New Delhi: Ministry of Health and Family Welfare).

Government of India (2011): 'Table 6.2.2 State/UT wise Number of Government Hospitals & Beds in Rural & Urban Areas (Including CHCs) In India (Provisional)', in 'Health Infrastructure' in *National Health Profile, 2011* (New Delhi: Central Bureau of Health Intelligence, Ministry of Health and Family Welfare).

Government of India (2004-5): *National Health Accounts 2004-05 (With Provisional Estimates from 2005–06 to 2008–09)*, (New Delhi: Ministry of Health and Family Welfare).

Gandy, M., (2005): 'Deadly Alliances: Death, Disease, and the Global Politics of Public Health', *PLoS Medicine*, Vol. 2 (1) e4: 9-11.

Gangolli, L.V., Ravi Duggal, Abhay Shukla (2005): *Review of Health care In India* (Mumbai: Centre for Enquiry into Health and Allied Themes, Research Centre of Anusandhan Trust), January.

High Level Expert Group (HLEG) (2011): 'Human Resources for Health', in *High Level Expert Group Report on Universal Health Coverage for India* (New Delhi: Planning Commission, Government of India), October, p. 140.

Hong, E. (2000): 'Globalisation and the Impact on Health: A Third World View', Third World Network, prepared for The Peoples' Health Assembly, December 4–8, 2000, Savar, Bangladesh.

John, M.D., S. J. Chander, N. Devadasan (2008): National Urban Health Mission: An Analysis of Strategies and Mechanisms for Improving Services for Urban Poor, Background Paper for National Workshop on Urban Health and Poverty, July 2-3, 2008, New Delhi; organized by Ministry of Housing and Urban Poverty Alleviation, Government of India. Available from http://www.academia.edu/855928/National_Urban_Health_Mission_An_analysis_of_strategies_and_mechanisms_ for_improving_services_for_urban_poor, accessed on January 7, 2014.

Jan Swasthya Abhiyan (2006): *Health System in India: Crisis & Alternatives, Towards the National Health Assembly II,* Booklet 2, October.

Jha, D.N. (2012): 'All India Institute of Medical Sciences Faces Exodus of Top Doctors'. *Times of India,* May 3. Available from http://articles.timesofindia.indiatimes.com/2012-05-03/delhi/31555155_1_faculty-association-voluntary-retirement-faculty-members Accessed on January 7, 2014.

Jan Swasthya Abhiyan (2007): 'New Technologies in Public Health – Who Pays and Who Benefits?' (first ed.), January.

Jan Swasthya Abhiyan (2006a): 'Globalization and Health', October.

Jan Swasthya Abhiyan (2006b): 'Health System in India: Crisis and Alternatives, Towards the National Health Assembly II', Booklet 2, October, p. 24.

Kim Jim Yong, (2013): 'World Bank Group President Jim Yong Kim's Speech at World Health Assembly: Poverty, Health and the Human Future', The World Bank. Available from http://www.worldbank.org/en/news/speech/2013/05/21/world-bank-group-president-jim-yong-kim-speech-at-world-health-assembly accessed on September 5, 2013.

Kaushik, M., A. Jaiswal , N. Shah, et al. (2008): 'High-End Physician Migration from India.', *Bull World Health Organ,* 86(1): 40-5.

Mehta, R., B. Gulshan, A.P. Singh, M. Khejriwal (2010): 'A Peek into the Future of Health care: Trends for 2010, Technopak Perspective: A Quarterly Report, pp. 45–58, quoted in *High Level Expert Group Report on Universal Health Coverage for India,* November, 2011 (New Delhi: Planning Commission).

Muralidharan, K., Nazmul Chaudhury, Jeffrey Hammer, et al. (2011): 'Is There a Doctor in the House? Medical Worker Absence in India,' Working Paper, Dept of Economics, Faculty of Arts and Sciences, Harvard University. Available from http://scholar.harvard.edu/files/kremer/files/is_there_a_doctor_in_the_house_-_12_april_2011.pdf accessed on January 6, 2014.

Macaulay, T.B. (1835): Minute on Indian Education. Delivered on February 3, 1835 in the British Parliament. Accessed at *h*ttp://www.columbia.edu/itc/mealac/pritchett/00generallinks/macaulay/txt_minute_education 1835.html accessed on September 7, 2013.

Mudaliar Committee (1959): Health Survey and Development Committee, Delhi: Government of India).

Maurya, A.K., A.K. Singh, M. Kumar. et al. (2013): 'Changing Patterns and Trends of Multidrug-Resistant Tuberculosis at Referral Centre in Northern India: A 4-Year Experience, *Indian Journal of Medical Microbiology*, Jan.–Mar., Vol. 31(1): 40-6, doi: 10.4103/0255-0857.108720.

Marriot, A. (2009): 'Blind Optimism Challenging the Myths about Private Health care in Poor Countries', Oxfam Briefing Paper 125, February.

Nandan D., K.S. Nair, and U. Datta (2007): 'Human Resources for Public Health in India: Issues and Challenges', *Health and Population – Perspectives and Issues,* Vol. 30(4): 230-242.

Perappadan, B.S., (2012): 'Private Hospitals Advertise at AIIMS to Recruit Doctors', *Hindu,* May 6. Available from http://www.thehindu.com/todays-paper/tp-national/private-hospitals-advertise-at-aiims-to-recruit-doctors/article3389387.ece and accessed on January 7, 2014.

Rao, M., K.D. Rao, A.K. Kumar, et al. (2011): 'Human Resources for Health in India', *Lancet,* February 12., Vol. 377(9765): 587-98.

Rao, K., A. Bhatnagar, P. Berman (2009): 'India's Health Workforce: Size, Composition and Distribution', in J. La Forgia and K. Rao (eds.) (New Delhi:World Bank/Public Health Foundation of India, India Health Beat).

Reserve Bank of India (2012-13): *Handbook of Statistics on Indian Economy, 2011-12.*

Reddy, K.S. (2012): 'Universal Health Coverage in India: The Time Has Come', *National Medical Journal of India,* Vol. 25 (2): 65-7.

Singh, Manmohan (2005): 'Of Oxford, Economics, Empire, and Freedom', *Hindu,* online edition dated July 10, 2005. Accessed at http://www.hindu.com/2005/07/10/stories/2005071002301000.htm on September 22, 2009.

Sidel, V.W. and R. Sidel (1973): 'Serve the People: Observations on Medicine in the People's Republic of China' (Boston: Beacon Press).

Sidel, R., and Sidel, V.W. (1982): 'The Health of China' (London: Zed Press).

Sokhey Committee, 1948: *Sub-Committee on National Health, National Planning Committee* (Bombay: Vora & Co.), p. 35.

Sathyamala, C., O. Mittal, R. Dasgupta, and R. Priya (2005): 'Polio Eradication Initiative in India: Deconstructing the GPEI', *Int J. Health Serv.,* Vol. 35 (2): 361-83.

Verma S.K. (1997): 'Fms Invitation To MNCs Raises Swadeshi Hackles', *Business Standard,* February 27. Accessed from http://www.business-standard.com/article/economy-policy/fms-invitation-to-mncs-raises-swadeshi-hackles-197022701116_1.html on March 31, 2015.

World Health Organization (WHO) (2010): *Global Atlas of the Health Workforce* (Geneva: WHO).

WHO (1978): 'Primary Health Care – Report of the International Conference on Primary Health Care, Alma-Ata, USSR, September 6-12, 1978', Geneva.

Yadav, K., P. Jarhyan , V. Gupta, et al. (2009): 'Revitalizing Rural Health Care Delivery: Can Rural Health Practitioners Be the Answer?', *Indian Journal of Community of Medicine,* January, Vol. 34(1): 3–5.

7

Socio-economic Inequalities and Health Outcomes in India

Introduction

In the 1980s, according to a Brazilian leader, the economic reforms and structural adjustment in his country led to a situation where 'the economy does well, but the people do poorly' (Goulet, 2002, 20). At the end of two decades of similar economic reforms in India, this statement is equally true for the majority of people in India. Structural adjustment policies have led to a widening of socio-economic inequities in society. This has implications for health outcomes among different social groups. We use data from the National Family Health Survey (NFHS) and other sources to discuss issues relating to health disparities based on class, caste and gender.

A Conceptual Framework for an Understanding of Equity

It is widely recognized that 'health outcomes' depend upon socio-economic factors, and inequalities lead to differences in health status among individuals or social groups. Braveman defined 'equity in health' as 'the absence of systematic disparities in health or in the major social determinants of health, between social groups who have different levels of underlying social advantage/ disadvantage, that is, different positions in a social hierarchy' (Braveman and Gruskin, 2003). Also, 'inequities in health systematically put groups of people who are already socially disadvantaged (for example, by virtue of being poor, female, and/ or members of a disenfranchised racial, ethnic or religious group) at further disadvantage with respect to their health; health being essential to well-being and to overcoming other effects of social disadvantage' (Braveman and Gruskin, 2003). The 'social group' could be a category based on a social characteristic such as socio-economic class, gender, race, ethnicity, religion and, in the Indian context, caste. This concept of 'equity in health' is in contrast to earlier attempts at measuring disparities in health simply between 'ungrouped individuals' (Murray et al., 1999; WHO, 2000).

Health equity implies that social and economic policies should be designed to bridge disparities in health between different social groups. With the state increasingly using market-guided mechanisms, there has been a skewed social development of different sections of society. While the upper and the upper middle classes have cornered the lion's share of social wealth, the lower classes have continued to remain disadvantaged.

Braveman draws a distinction between 'health equity' and 'equality in health'. 'Health equity' deals with processes that determine the distribution of resources necessary for health and the processes that lead to systematic disparities in health or social determinants of health between different social groups. On the other hand, 'equality/inequality in health' implies measurement of appropriate health indicators for different social groups which facilitate comparison between these social groups (Braveman, 2003). Thus, while 'health equity' facilitates a judgement of health policies and social processes as being conducive or otherwise to achieving greater equality of health between different social groups, 'equality in health' helps in monitoring the impact of health policies. The levels of health enjoyed by the most advantaged groups could be a benchmark of what is possible for the other groups.

Socio-economic Inequities

The major socio-economic inequalities that influence health outcomes include those due to income or social class, caste, gender, rural-urban setting and geographical region. There is considerable interaction between these factors, with additive effects. Thus, health impairment for a lower class person belonging to a low caste may be much greater than that for a lower class person of a high caste. Persons belonging to the scheduled castes (SC) and scheduled tribes (ST), and in some cases 'other backward castes', often live in relatively inaccessible areas and are more likely to be poor (Nayar,

2007). Data from the 52nd round of National Sample Survey (NSS) on deciles of consumption expenditure (Table 1) show that 65 per cent of SC and ST households live below the poverty line, are uneducated, and live in rural areas (SASHD and SASFP, 2004). The lower castes are thus disadvantaged because they have no resources to spend on health care, are less educated, and live in rural areas where they have limited access to health services.

Table 1: Socio-economic Correlates of Poverty

Income Decile	*Proportion of SC/ST (%)*	*Proportion with Less Than Primary Education (%)*	*Proportion Residing in Rural Areas (%)*
1	52.6	84.0	82.7
2	47.4	79.9	80.6
3	41.1	75.9	77.8
4	38.2	72.6	74.0
5	33.2	68.0	69.6
6	30.9	63.8	64.5
7	27.2	58.9	58.7
8	24.0	53.6	52.5
9	21.2	48.7	46.0
10	13.9	41.5	37.2

Source: Gupta I., Datta A. Inequities in Health and Health care in India: Can the Poor Hope for a Respite. IEG Discussion Paper Series No. 80/2003, Institute of Economic Growth, Delhi. SC: Scheduled Castes ST: Scheduled Tribes

Our health policies place an emphasis on the allopathic system over indigenous systems of medicine, and on curative over preventive medicine. There is also a concentration of medical facilities in urban centres with an overwhelming neglect of rural areas and dominance of for-profit private health care over public facilities (Gangoli et al., 2005; Banerji, 1979; Baru et al., 2010). Policy-makers place less emphasis on improving access to health care for the marginalized sections of the population.

The failure to recognize links between different forms of socio-economic disparity leads to ineffective implementation of various poverty-alleviation as well as social and health programmes (Iyer et al., 2008). For example, it is not uncommon for village *anganwadis* or immunization booths to be located in upper caste localities, or an auxillary nurse-midwife to visit only upper caste homes, neglecting the lower castes. There is therefore a need for more public investment in quality health care in rural areas, an emphasis on providing preventive health services to the disadvantaged groups, and a sensitization of health services and health care providers to the barriers faced by the SC/ST groups and the poor in accessing health services, administrative steps to ensure equitable compliance, and an institution of measures to ensure participation of marginalized social groups in poverty-alleviation programmes. These small steps will help increase awareness of equity issues and will also help create an atmosphere conducive to larger efforts such as a major redistribution of resources.

Health Disparities by Social Class

Social class is widely recognized as an important determinant of health. Economic deprivation means denial of access to resources required for a life of dignity. Marginalization of such deprived populations leads to social disintegration and has implications for health. The theory of 'social support' has documented the effect of social integration on health (Cassel, 1976). Wilkinson has argued that the relative distribution of income is more important to the health of people than absolute deprivation of income (Wilkinson, 1992).

Several studies have shown a strong association between income inequality and mortality. Of these, the *Black Report*, prepared by a Research Working Group on Inequalities in Health in Great Britain has historical importance (Townsend et al., 1988). It found large differences in morbidity and mortality that favoured the higher social classes and were not being redressed by the health or social services (BMJ editorial, 1980). Other studies have reached similar conclusions (Ben-Shlomo et al., 1996; Kaplan et al., 1996). Kennedy et al. found a direct effect of income inequality on total mortality in a population (Kennedy et al., 1996). However, in India, no class-based data on health are available.

Globalization has led to the widening of various socio-economic disparities around the world. In India too, it has led to increasing social, regional and rural-urban disparities (Baru et al., 2010; National Coordination Committee, 2006). The Arjun Sen Gupta Committee report on unorganized labour reported that 77 per cent Indians live on less than Rs. 20 a day (Sengupta et al., 2008). This notwithstanding, the welfare sectors such as education and health have been increasingly opened to the for-profit private sector. This was at a time when the gross domestic product (GDP) growth rates had consistently been above 7 per cent and had even touched 9 per cent. It has been calculated that poverty has actually increased in India during the period between 1993-4 and 2004-5, despite official claims to the contrary. Adverse changes in income distribution in most states have offset the beneficial effects of economic growth during this period (Ravi, 2009). The poverty in rural areas has increased and has led to increasing disparities in access to health-care (Baru et al., 2010) as also health outcomes.

The NFHS-II data show that the infant mortality rate for the poorest 20 per cent of the population was 2.5-times higher than that for the richest 20 per cent (IIPS and ORC, 2000). Further, a child born in a tribal belt was 1.5 times more likely to die before his/her fifth birthday (IIPS and ORC, 2000). A person from the poorest quintile of the population, despite greater health problems, is 6 times less likely to access hospitalization than a person from the richest quintile. This means that the poor are unable to afford and access hospitalization in a very large proportion of illness episodes, even when it is necessary. The delivery of a mother from the poorest quintile of the population is over 6 times less likely to be attended by a medically trained person than the delivery of a well-off mother, from the richest quintile of the population. A tribal mother is over 12-times less likely to be delivered by a medically trained person (IIPS and ORC, 2000). A tribal woman is 1.5-times more likely to suffer the consequences of chronic malnutrition compared to women from other social categories. A World Bank study published in 2001, quoted by Mukhopadhaya, found that the poor-rich risk ratio is 2.5 for infant mortality, 2.8 for under-5 mortality, 1.7 for childhood underweight, and 2 for total fertility rate (World Bank, 2001). These figures bring to the fore not only the unequal distribution of resources and its effect on public health parameters but also the intersection between caste, class, and ethnicity.

An analysis of NFHS-3 data shows that health inequalities increased when rising average income levels of the population are accompanied by rising income inequalities (Joe et al., 2008). Table 2 shows the trends in child malnutrition in India from 1975-9 to

2004-5 (Deaton and Dreze, 2009). Over 50 per cent of children in India were underweight and stunted in 2004-5, while the proportion of severely underweight and stunted was as high as 18 and 25 per cent, respectively. While there has been a major decline, India still has a very high proportion of malnourished children (Table 3) and is placed below even Afghanistan. According to the National Nutrition Monitoring Bureau (NNMB) data (2002) (weight for age), 94.5 per cent children in the age group of 6-9 years, and 96.1 per cent children in the age group of 10-13 years were suffering from mild-to-severe malnutrition (NNMB, 2002).

Table 2: Changes in Nutritional Parameters of Children Over Time

Parameter	*Proportion (%) of Undernourished Children*					*Percentage Decline*
	1975-9	*1988-90*	*1996-7*	*2000-1*	*2004-5*	*(1974-5 to 2004-5)*
Weight for age (underweight)						
Below 2 SD	77	69	62	60	55	29
Below 3 SD	37	27	23	21	18	51
Height for age (stunting)						
Below 2 SD	79	65	58	49	52	34
Below 3 SD	53	37	29	26	25	53
Weight for height (wasting)						
Below 2 SD	18	20	19	23	15	17
Below 3 SD	2.9	2.5	2.5	3.1	2.4	17

Source: Deaton and Dreze, 2009.

Table 3: Countries with Highest Proportion of Malnourished Children

Country	*Proportion of Children Underweight (%)*
Nepal	48.3
Bangladesh	47.5
India	46.7
Timor-Leste	45.8
Yemen	45.6
Burundi	45.1
Madagascar	41.9
Sudan	40.7
Lao (People's Democratic Republic)	40.4
Niger	40.1
Eritrea	39.6
Afghanistan	39.3

Reproduced from Deaton and Dreze, 2009. Figures apply to the most recent year for which data are available within the reference period. There is a significant margin of error for individual countries

Similarly, despite a 41 and 31 per cent decline in the proportion of men and women, respectively, with a body mass index (BMI) <18.5, from 1975-9 to 2004-5, the proportion for women in India with BMI <18.5 is higher than that in sub-Saharan countries such as Rwanda, Malawi, Zimbabwe, Gabon, etc. (Deaton and Dreze, 2009). Interestingly, Baru et al. have shown that the rate of decline of infant mortality and under-5 mortality decreased in the years when economic reforms were implemented (Baru et al., 2010).

The increasing out-of-pocket expenditure on health during the past two decades has contributed to the increase in number of people below the poverty line (from 3.25 per cent of the population in 1999-2000 (Bonu et al., 2007; Garg and Karan, 2005) to 3.5 per cent of the population in 2005-6; an additional 32 million people. (Dreze and Sen, 21997).

Income and social gradients are also seen across diseases. Acute diarrhoeal diseases (ADD) are among the *principal* killers of children in India and follow a social gradient (Siddiqi, 2007). Analysis of data on cholera from Delhi shows that there is a gradient from planned colonies to slums; and among low-income colonies, from 'legal' to 'illegal' (Dasgupta, 2004 a; Dasgupta, 2004 b). The notion of legality, especially in the context of urban areas, means entitlement to access safe drinking water and healthier living conditions, which may be denied to illegal colonies.

A study meticulously documented the impact of economic status on maternal and child health among the residents of slum localities in Mumbai. It showed that the rate of marriage and conception in adolescents was less among women of a higher socio-economic quartile group (odds ratio 0.74, 95 per cent CI 0.690.79, and 0.82, 0.78-0.87, respectively). It also found that as the socio-economic status increased, there was a tendency to rely less on public sector health care (0.75, 0.70-0.79) for antenatal care and for institutional delivery (0.66, 0.61-0.71). Home deliveries were 5-times higher in the poorest group compared to the least poor group (0.17, 0.10-0.27) and deliveries in public sector facilities were about four times less likely in the least poor group in comparison to the poor group (0.27, 0.21-0.35). Higher socio-economic status meant lower prevalence of low birth weight (0.91, 0.85-0.97). The neonatal mortality rates also fell, though non-significantly as socio-economic status increased (0.88, 0.71-1.08) (More et al., 2009).

Various rounds of National Sample Surveys have shown that a higher percentage of the poor do not seek care when ill (World Bank, 2001). Also, a much lower percentage of the poor seek institutional care. In the case of institutional deliveries too, the poorest 20 per cent have only 100 institutional deliveries per 1,000 live-births compared to almost 700 deliveries for the richest 20 per cent. Looking at the total illness episodes treated during the past 15 days, the poorest 20 per cent obtained treatment three times less than the richest 20 per cent. The difference in the hospitalization rates was six times between the rich and the poor, even though it is the poor who fall ill more often and are in need of hospitalization (Misra et al., 2003). Inability to access health care due to poverty and high out-of-pocket expenditure worsens health outcomes for poorer households. It has been estimated that over 20 million Indians are pushed below the poverty line every year because of out-of-pocket spending on health care (Mudur, 2004). With private health care having acquired a commanding position in health-care delivery, health services are increasingly skewed towards an urban bias, tertiary level health services, with profitability overriding equality, and rationality of care often taking a back seat.

The declines in parameters such as infant mortality rate, under-5 mortality, maternal mortality, and different measures of malnutrition, etc. that have taken place are a result of technological interventions put into operation in programme mode, e.g. vaccination campaigns, maternal and child health and reproductive health interventions, water and sanitation campaigns, etc.

There has been no change in policy to redistribute societal resources to decrease socio-economic inequities. A persistent decline in the calories consumed by different household consumption categories has been documented in successive NSSO surveys, resulting in a rise in poverty as measured by the minimum nutritional criterion. The Tendulkar Committee appointed by the Planning Commission to determine the levels of poverty in India has sought to unpeg the old nutritional criterion as a determinant of poverty (GOI, 2009). Rising poverty, improper nutrition, and inability to access health care due to its increasing commercialization and privatization have put into jeopardy the gains made so far. India was placed at 134 among 182 countries in the United Nation's *Human Development Index 2009* in the category of 'medium human development'. We are nowhere near Brazil, China, Mexico, and South Africa (UNDP, 2009).[1]

Health Disparities by Caste

In India, class is not the only factor for health-related inequities. Caste and class inequities often go together. As mentioned above, the 'lower' castes are also lower economic classes, and the trajectories of health outcome indicators across caste groups and classes are similar. Table 4 shows the distribution of various health indicators according to the NFHS-3 data and follow a similar gradient across castes/tribes and economic class by wealth index (IIPS and Macro International, 2007). It can be seen that as with lower class, the lower castes and the tribes have much poorer health outcomes.

Mohindra et al. studied the impact of caste and socio-economic status on women's health in Kerala, a state with generally good health standards and progressive policies. They showed that both caste and socioeconomic status were associated with inequality in health and also accentuated their mutual effect. Interestingly, the higher 'caste' had a cushioning effect on the adverse effects of lower socio-economic status on the health of poor people of higher castes (Mohindra et al., 2006). These results reinforce the need for policy-makers to be sensitive to caste issues relating to health.

Heath Disparities by Gender

The nature of health problems faced by men and women and their health needs differ. In India, mortality is higher among women in all age-groups, negating the biological advantage that women naturally possess. The reproductive health needs of men and women are different. How are these differences to be understood? Can they be explained only on the basis of the biological differences between sexes, or factors such as poverty, education, etc.? Can these differences be addressed by similar policy initiatives for men and women or is there a need for a more nuanced approach specifically

Table 4: Health Outcome Indicators Disaggregated by Caste/Tribe and Economic Class

Factor/ and category	*Infant mortality rate (per 1000 live-births)*	*Under-5 mortality (per 1000 live-births)*	*Chronic malnutrition (low height for age) in children under 5 (% of children below 2SD)*	*Anaemia in children 6-59 months of age (%)*	*15-49 year-olds with anaemia*		*15-45 year-olds with BMI<18.5*		*Deliveries in health facilities (%)*	*Households covered by health scheme/ insurance(%)*
					Women (%)	*Men (%)*	*Women (%)*	*Men (%)*		
Caste/tribe										
SC	66.4	88.1	53.9	72.2	58.3	26.6	41.1	39.1	32.9	3.3
ST	62.1	95.7	53.9	76.8	68.5	39.6	46.6	41.3	17.7	2.6
OBC	56.6	72.8	48.8	70.3	54.4	22.3	35.7	34.6	37.7	3.8
Others	48.9	59.2	40.7	63.8	51.3	20.9	29.4	28.9	51.0	7.8
Wealth index										
Lowest	70.4	100.5	59.9	76.4	64.3	37.9	51.5	48.3	12.7	0.1
Second	68.5	89.6	54.3	73.6	60.3	30.2	46.3	42.4	23.5	0.7
Middle	58.3	71.9	48.9	69.3	56.0	24.8	38.3	37.4	39.2	2.2
Fourth	44.0	51.2	40.8	64.8	52.2	18.8	28.9	29.6	57.9	5.1
Highest	29.2	33.8	25.3	56.2	46.1	14.2	18.2	19.1	83.7	16.4

Source: Compiled from *National Family Health Survey* (NFHS-3), 2005–06, India, Volume I.38. SD = Standard Deviation BMI = Body Mass Index; SC = Scheduled Caste; ST = Scheduled Tribe; OBC = Other Backward Castes.

relating to men and women as separate categories?

The term 'sex' refers to the biological differences between men and women, whereas 'gender' refers to 'socially constructed roles and responsibilities that women and men carry out which are differentially and hierarchically located and valued in various cultures' (Lingam and Pitre, 2008). The differential valuation of roles played by men and women, which is determined by the prevalent values and belief systems, can be seen in society across institutions, e.g. marriage, family, communities, caste, class, and the like. Such a differential valuation often places women at a disadvantage vis-à-vis men and leads to their subordination in society (Lingam and Pitre, 2008).

This has important implications for women's health issues. In India, the vast differences between health outcomes among men and women are often attributed to inequities in education and/or income. However, the maternal mortality rate in Vietnam was 160 with a per capita GDP of US$ 1,860, whereas in India it was 407 with a per capita GDP of US$ 2,248 (Kaur, 2005). Similarly, economically prosperous states such as Punjab and Haryana have sex ratios of 874 and 861, respectively, while it is 972 in Odisha, a much poorer state (Kaur, 2005). These data reinforce the need for a gender perspective to health.

There is empirical evidence on the adverse impact of gender on women's health. According to NFHS-3 (2006-07), 46.6 per cent of urban and 51 per cent of rural women aged 15-49 years are anaemic (Fig. 1); these proportions are much higher than those for men (Lingam and Pitre, 2008b).

Similarly, both inpatient and outpatient expenditure on health of women is much lower than that for men in all age groups even in a state like Maharashtra (Tables 5 and 6).

Table 5: Average Medical Expenditure on Inpatient Treatment by Gender, Maharashtra 1995-6 and 2004

Characteristic	*Mean Medical Expenditure on Inpatient Care (in Rs)*					
	1995-96			*2004*		
	Public	*Private*	*Total*	*Public*	*Private*	*Total*
Men	1,572	4,845	3,845	2,948	9,642	7,960
Women	910	3,451	2,549	2,265	8,444	6,794

Source: Lingam and Pitre, 2008b

Fig. 1: Anaemia Among Ever-Married and Pregnant Women and Ever-Married Men

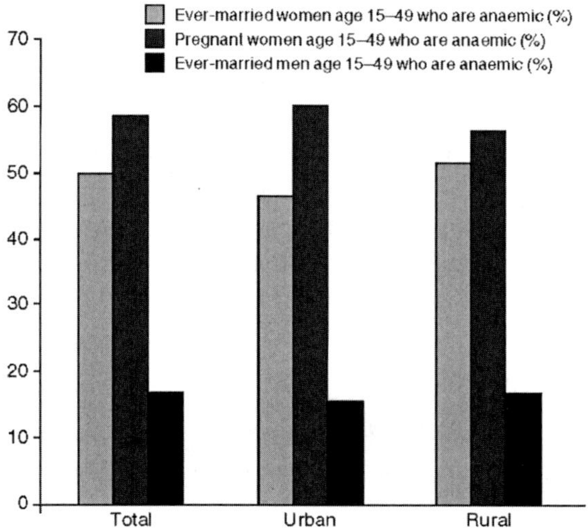

Source: Reproduced from Lingam L., Pitre, A. (2008a)

Table 6: Average Medical Expenditure for Non-Hospitalized Treatment Per Ailing Person During a Period of 15 Days by Age and Gender, Maharashtra 2004

Age (years)	*Average Expenditure (in Rs.)*		
	Male	*Female*	*Total*
0-15	251	166	213
16-39	318	228	267
40-59	336	297	313
>60	313	246	279

Source: Reproduced from Lingam and Pitre, A. (2008b)

There is an urgent need to sensitize health care professionals about gender analysis tools, to help them understand the differences in health outcomes between men and women, in an attempt to bridge the gender gap. The term 'gender analysis' implies a 'systematic examination of the roles, relations, and the processes that focus on the imbalance of power, wealth, workload opportunities and constraints as experienced by women and men in a given community'. Gender gaps in health result from the inequality in decision-making leading to unequal access to resources for women and girls compared to men and boys.

Conclusion

Socio-economic disparities are an important determinant of health outcomes. No longer can we ignore health disparities. We, as health care professionals, need to ensure a more equitable health-care system for the poor and disadvantaged. Whether the current obsession with 'universal health care', in the mould of insurance based delivery of health services, is the answer only time will tell. However, authors apprehend that this will lead to more queries than answers.

REFERENCES

Braveman, P., and S. Gruskin (2003): 'Defining Equity in Health', *Journal of Epidemiology and Community Health,* Vol. 57: 254-8.

Braveman, P., A. (2003): 'Monitoring Equity in Health and Health care: A Conceptual Framework', *Journal of Health Population and Nutrition,* 21:181-92.

Banerji, D. (1979): 'The Place of Indigenous and Western Systems of Medicine in the Health Services of India', *Social Science and Medicine Part A: Medical Psychology and Medical Sociology,* 15A (2):109-14.

Baru, R., A. Achary, S. Acharya , A.K. Shiva Kumar, et al. (2010): 'Inequities in Access to Health Services in India: Caste, Class and Region', *Economic and Political Weekly,* 45: 49-58.

BMJ Editorial (1980): 'Equalities and Inequalities in Health', *British Medical Journal,* Vol. 281: 762-3.

Ben-Shlomo, Y., I.R. White, and M. Marmot (1996): 'Does the Variation in the Socio-economic Characteristics of an Area Affect Mortality? *British Medical Journal,* Vol. 312: 1013-14.

Bonu, S., I. Bhushan, and D.H. Peters (2007): 'Incidence, Intensity and Correlates of Catastrophic Out-of-pocket Hhealth Payments in India,' ERD Working Paper No. 102, Asian Development Bank, Manila.

Cassel, J. (1976): 'The Contribution of the Social Environment to Host Resistance:, Fourth Wade Hampton Frost Lecture', *Am J. Epidemiol,* Vol. 104: 107-23.

Deaton, A., and J. Dreze (2009): 'Food and nutrition in India: Facts and Interpretations', *Economic and Political Weekly,* Vol. 44: 42-65.

Dreze, J., and A. Se (eds) (1997): *Indian Development: Selected Regional Perspectives,* Oxford University Press, New Delhi.

Dasgupta, P. and R. Dasgupta (2004): Economic Value of Safe Water for the Infrastructurally Disadvantaged Urban Household: A Case Study in Delhi, India, *Water Resources Research,* Vol. 40: W11401.

Dasgupta, R. (2004): 'Cholera in Delhi: Time Trends and its Determinants', Doctoral Thesis Centre of Social Medicine and Community Health, Jawaharlal Nehru University, New Delhi.

Goulet, D. (2002): 'What is a Just Economy in a Globalized World?' *Intenational Journal of Social Economics,* Vol. 29 (1-2): 10–25.

Gangolli, L.V., R. Duggal, and A. Shukla (2005):, *Review of Health care in India,* Mumbai, Centre for Enquiry into Health and Allied Themes, Research Centre of Anusandhan Trust. Available at http:// www.cehat.org/publications /PDf%20files/r51.pdf and accessed on June 12, 2010.

Garg, C. and A.K. Karan (2005): Health and Millennium Development Goal 1: Reducing Out-of-pocket Expenditures to Reduce Income Poverty—Evidence for India, EQUITAP Project, Working Paper No. 15, Institute of Health Policy, Colombo.

GOI (Government of India) (2009): 'Report of the Expert Group to Review the Methodology for Estimation of Poverty.' Planning Commission, November, p. 14.

Iyer, A., G. Sen, and P. Ostlin (2008): 'The Intersections of Gender and Class in Health Status and Health care.' *Global Public Health,* Vol. 3 (1):13-24. doi: 10.1080/17441690801892174.

International Institute for Population Sciences (IIPS) and ORC Macro (2000): *National Family Health Survey (NFHS-2), India 1998-99,* Mumbai, India and Maryland, USA, October.

International Institute for Population Sciences (IIPS) and Macro International (2007): *National Family Health Survey (NFHS-3), 2005-06: India:* Vol. I, Mumbai: IIPS. Compiled from Tables: 7.2 (p. 182), 8.12 (p. 208), 10.1 (p. 270), 10.12 (p. 289), 10.22.1 (p. 304), 10.22.2 (p. 306), 10. 24. 1 (p. 311), 10. 24. 2 (p. 312).

Joe, W., U.S. Mishra, and K. Navaneetham (2008): 'Health Inequality in India: Evidence from NFHS 3, *Economic and Political Weekly,* Vol. 43: 41-8.

Kaplan, G.A., E.R., Pamuk, J.W. Lynch, et al. (1996): 'Inequality in Income and Mortality in the United States: Analysis of Mortality and Potential Pathways', *British Medical Journal,* Vol. 312: 999-1003.

Kennedy, B.P., I. Kawachi, and D. Prothrow-Stith (1996): 'Income Distribution and Mortality: Cross Sectional Ecological Study of the Robin Hood Index in the United States', *British Medical Journal,* Vol. 312: 1004-7.

Kaur, M. (2005): 'Mainstreaming Gender in Health', *Indian Journal of*

Community Medicine, Vol. 30: 75-7.

Lingam, L., and A. Pitre (2008): 'Gender Inequities in Health Access and Outcomes' in N. Sardeshpande and A. Shukla (eds.) (2008): *'A Report on Health Inequities in Maharashtra',* SATHI (Support for Advocacy and Training into Health Initiatives), in collaboration with CEHAT and TISS, Pune, Maharashtra, 75-94. Available at www.sathicehat.org/uploads/Equity Watch/him.pdf, accessed on April 9, 2012.

Lingam, L., and A. Pitre (2008): 'Annexure VII: Health care Utilization Tables', In N. Sardeshpande and A. Shukla (eds), *'A Report on Health Inequities in Maharashtra',* SATHI (Support for Advocacy and Training into Health Initiatives), in collaboration with CEHAT and TISS, Pune, Maharashtra, 110. Available at www.sathicehat.org/uploads/ Equity Watch/him.pdf, accessed on April 9, 2012.

Murray, C., J.E.E. Gakidou, and J. Frenk (1999): 'Health Inequalities and Social Group Differences: What Should We Measure?', *Bulletin of World Health Organization,* Vol. 77: 537-43.

More, N.S., U. Bapat , S. Das S., et al. (2009): 'Inequalities in Maternity Care and Newborn Outcomes: One-Year Surveillance of Births in Vulnerable Slum Communities in Mumbai', *International Journal Equity Health,* Vol. 8: 21.

Misra, R., R. Chatterjee , and S. Rao (2003): *India Health Report,* Oxford University Press, New Delhi.

Mudur, G. (2004): 'Inadequate Regulations Undermine India's Health care', *BMJ,* Vol. 328: 124.

Mohindra, K.S., S. Haddad, and D., Narayana (2006): 'Women's Health in a Rural Community in Kerala, India: Do Caste and Socio-economic Position Matter?' *Journal of Epidemiology and Community Health,* Vol. 60: 1020-6.

Nayar, K.R. (2007): 'Social Exclusion, Caste and Health: A Review Based on the Social Determinants Framework', *Indian Journal Medicine Research,* 126: 355-63.

National Coordination Committee (2006): 'Globalization and Health.' Jan Swasthya Abhiyan, October 2006.

National Nutrition Monitoring Bureau (2002): *'Diet and Nutritional Status of Rural Population,' NNMB Tech Report No. 21*: National Institute of Nutrition, Hyderabad.

Ravi, C. (2009): Impact of Globalization and Recession on Social and Economic Inequalities in India. Paper for Conference on 'The Impact of the Global Economic Situation on Poverty and Sustainable development in Asia and the Pacific', September 28-30, 2009, Hanoi. Available at http://www.adb.org/documents/events/2009/Poverty-Social-Development/globalization-impact-on-inequality-in-

India-Ravi-paper.pdf, accessed on November 4, 2009.

SASHD, SASFP (2004): *'India-Private Health Services for the Poor'* (Policy Note, May 2004) Available at http://www.sasnet.lu.se/EASAS papers/11IsmailRadwan.pdf, accessed on November 4, 2009.

Sengupta, A., K.P. Kannan, G. Raveendran (2008): 'India's Common People: Who Are They, How Many Are They and How Do They Live? *Economic and Political Weekly*, Vol. 43 (11): 49 – 63.

Siddiqi, A., L.G. Irwin and C. Hertzman (2007): *'Total Environment Assessment Model for Early Child Development: Evidence Report for the Commission on Social Determinants of Health'*, Commission on Social Determinants of Health, World Health Organization, Geneva, Switzerland.

Townsend, P., N. Davidson, and M. Whitehead, (1988): *Inequalities in Health: The Black Report and the Health Divide,* Penguin, Harmondsworth.

UNDP (2009): 'Human movement: Snapshots and Trends.' In: *Human Development Report 2009*, United Nations Development Programme, pp. 145-46.

World Health Organization (WHO) (2000): *The World Health report 2000—Health Systems: Improving Performance,* (Geneva: World Health Organization), p. 205.

Wilkinson, R.G. (1992): 'Income Distribution and Life Expectancy', *British Medical Journal,* Vol. 304: 165-8.

World Bank (2001), quoted in Alok Mukhopadhyay (2011): Effective Social Determinants of Health Approach in India Through Community Mobilization, Voluntary Health Association of India. Draft background paper 9, World Conference on Social Determinants of Health, Rio de Janeiro, Brazil, October 19-21. Available from www.who.int/entity/.../resources/draft_background_paper9_ india.pdf and accessed on April 9, 2012.

8

The Play of Religion in the Delivery of Rural Health Care: Impressions from Mewat District in Haryana*

Introduction

Created on April 4, 2005, Mewat is the twentieth district of Haryana state which is located barely 50 kms from the Delhi International Airport. Carved out of parts of Gurgaon district of the state, Mewat district lies in the Mewat region that spans Mewat and Palwal districts of Haryana, parts of Alwar, Bharatpur, and Dholpur districts of Rajasthan and Mathura in Uttar Pradesh. The region has a distinct ethno-cultural identity and derives its name from the Meo Muslims of the region who constitute the predominant population (more than 60 per cent) group. They converted to Islam from Hinduism under the influence of Sufi Islam during the reign of the Tughlak dynasty in the 14th century (MDA, 2011a).

The district comprises five blocks: Nuh, Tauru, Firozpur Jirkha, Nagina, and Punhana. The district headquarters are located at Nuh town. According to the 2001 census, the total population of the Mewat region of Haryana (including Hatin block of Palwal district)

---

* The findings regarding the district discussed here were made by me as part of the field study of the district health system of Mewat in 2010 when pursuing a Masters in Public Health Course from the Centre for Social Medicine and Community Health at Jawaharlal Nehru University, New Delhi. It is also acknowledged that things may well have improved in the district since the time of the visit, but subsequent improvements do not prejudice the findings of this report which beget our attention and concern in as much as these reflect the realities of Indian society.

Table 1: Comparison of Population and Household Characteristics of Mewat District with Those of Haryana State

Characteristics	*Mewat*		*State level characteristics (where it is differently worded than district level characteristics)*	*Haryana*	
	Total (%)	*Rural (%)*		*Total (%)*	*Rural (%)*
Total literate population (Age 7 +)	53.6	51.8		73.4	70.2
Literate male population (Age 7+)	72.9	71.8		-	-
Literate female population (Age 7+)	33.7	31.3		55.7[1]	-
HH with electricity connection	78.8	77.0		92.4	90.5
HH with access to toilet facility	16.2	12.2		56.3	45.3
Use piped drinking water	35.1	31.6	Improved source of drinking water[2]	96.0	94.7
Use LPG for cooking	4.5	1.4		-	-
Live in pucca house	34.6	30.9		58.0	48.7
Have a BPL card	24.5	24.6		8.74[1]	-
Own agricultural land	53.7	56.7		-	-
Own a motorized vehicle	21.2	20.0		-	-
Standard of living					
Low	64.0	67.3	Lowest wealth quintile	1.7	2.2
Medium	24.1	24.4	-	-	
High	11.9	8.3	Highest wealth quintile	37.8	26.7

Source: Figures have been taken from Haryana State Report, Progress of NRHM, MOHFW, New Delhi.Improved source of drinking water in DLHS – 3 included: piped into dwelling, piped to yard/plot, public tap/stand pipe/hand pump/tube well/bore-well/covered well or spring, tanker, cart with small tank and bottled water.

Compiled from the fact-sheets for Mewat and Haryana of the District Level Household Survey – 3 [GOI, 2007-08 a].

Note: The figures given in this table are inclusive of Hatin block which was subsequently separated from Mewat district and formed part of a new district, Palwal.

was 9,93,617, of which 46,122 (4.64 per cent) was urban, while 9,47,495 (95.36 per cent) was rural (MDA, 2011 a). This is in sharp contrast to the fact that the district is situated alongside Gurgaon, known for its trendy shopping malls, residential complexes, and skyscrapers; as also Faridabad which is another industrial hub and a prosperous urban centre. Of the total of 1,42,822 households, 53,125 (37 per cent) were below the official poverty line compared to 8.74 and 26.1 for Haryana and India respectively (MDA, 2011b). The average family size in the region was 7.5 (Government of India, 2009). All the corresponding details were not available from the 2011 census figures; however, the total population, rural and urban, of Mewat were 1,089,263,965,157 (88.61 per cent) and 1,24,106 (11.39 per cent) respectively (*Census of India*, 2013).

General Development Profile of the District

Table 1 below, which gives the comparison of socio-economic indicators of Mewat with those of Haryana State testifies to the socio-economic backwardness of Mewat. Tables 2 and 3 provide a comparison of selected health indicators of Mewat and Haryana.

Table 2: Maternal Health Undices from DLHS – 3 Survey

Parameter	*Mewat*	*Haryana*
Mothers registered in the first trimester when they were pregnant with last live birth/still birth (%)	17.4	55.1
Mothers who received at least 3 ante-natal care visits during the last pregnancy (%)	16.4	51.9
Mothers who received at least one TT injection when they were pregnant with their last live birth/stillbirth (%)	52.6	86.1
Institutional births (%)	14.8	46.9
Delivery at home assisted by a doctor/nurse /LHV/ ANM (%)	1.7	6.5
Mothers who received post natal care within 48 hours of delivery of their last child (%)	33.5	N.A.

Source: Compiled from the fact sheets for Mewat and Haryana of the District Level Household Survey – 3 (GOI, 2007-08).

Table 3: Child Health Indicators in Mewat

Parameter	*Mewat*	*Haryara*
Children (12-23 months) fully immunized (BCG, 3 doses each of DPT, and polio and one dose of measles) (%)	12.2	59.6
Children (9-35 months) who have received at least one dose of Vit. A (%)	8.1	46.3
Treatment of childhood diseases (children under 3 years based on last two surviving children)		
Children with diarrhoea in the last two weeks who received ORS (%)	7.6	31.7
Children with diarrhoea in the last two weeks who were given treatment (%)	74.8	82.0
Child feeding practices (children under 3 years)		
Children breastfed within one hour of birth (%)	7.6	17.4
Children (age 6 months above) exclusively breastfed (%)[1]	0.9	5.7
Children (6-24 months) who received solid or semi-solid food while still being breastfed (%).	72.7	74.1

[1] Children who were given nothing but breast milk till the survey date.
Source: Compiled from the fact sheets for Mewat and Haryana of the District Level Household Survey – 3 (GOI, 2007 – 8).

The Social, Economic, Political, and Cultural Context of Health in Mewat

One of the cardinal principles of public health is that the health of the people and the health systems ought to be studied in their social, economic, political, and cultural context. Even though there is little dispute about such a need, the same set of empirical findings relating to these contexts can be interpreted very differently by government planners, health personnel, activists working in the field, and the common people themselves. This can lead to a varied diagnosis of what ails the public health system and the interventions necessary to correct these. This makes it incumbent upon us to thoroughly document the social, economic, political, and cultural context of the people.

The Delhi-Alwar highway is the major highway passing through the district. A drive along it from Delhi gave an impression that development is just about beginning to occur in Mewat, i.e. over 60 years after India's independence. The highway was then being broadened into four lanes and was undergoing major repair work all along the route. The journey along the road could by no means be described as comfortable and yet, if the people of the region are to be believed, the condition of the highway, as it was then, was immensely better than it was even a year or two earlier. The implication very clearly is that for a patient suffering any surgical or medical emergency in this district, which does not have a single multi-specialty hospital worth its name, this road could well be the difference between life and death, because such a patient has invariably to be taken either to Delhi/Gurgaon or Alwar for medical attention.

A drive down the Delhi-Mathura highway or the Delhi-Jaipur or Delhi-Chandigarh highway, which are the other major highways connecting Delhi to the adjoining districts of Haryana give the impression that Haryana is not just an agricultural state but also a state that is rapidly industrializing, with towns that are ostensibly prosperous and where big business is rapidly spreading its tentacles. The picture of Mewat is in sharp contrast to this. Crossing from Gurgaon into Mewat is like a precipitous fall from a high cliff into a deep gorge. The dusty towns of Mewat, including the district headquarter of Nuh, provide a sharp contrast to the high rise malls, office complexes, and luxury apartments of Gurgaon which are barely 30 kms from Nuh. There was not even a single industrial shed along the Delhi-Alwar highway within Mewat. The only imposing structures that one found were the large mosques that dot the region with fair regularity and, unlike the rest of Haryana, it was not uncommon to find thatched katchha mud) houses in the villages along the route.

Passing through the towns along the highway one could typically find long lines of trucks parked on either side of the road and a number of auto-workshops. This was quite in consonance with a later finding that truck driving is one of the important accessory professions for the men folk of the region. Another sight that was fairly common in the villages along the way was that of small girls and women carrying containers of water. Mewat is a region acutely short of potable water.

The reasons for the backwardness of Mewat are multi-factorial; it is important to understand them in order to get a proper idea of the state of the health services and the health problems of the people of the region. Among the various factors that have been held to be responsible for the backwardness of the district are scarcity of adequate water resources for human consumption and agriculture, low productivity of agriculture and farm animals in the region, lack of education, the superstitions and religious conservatism of the people, large family sizes, political neglect of the region, poor health of the people, and a soaring crime rate. It needs to be mentioned here that all these factors are not simply additive in their effect, but operate as a complex interacting whole which is not amenable to straightjacketed technocratic solutions.

I shall restrict myself here to enumerating the empirical facts regarding each of these factors.

The Water Crisis of Mewat

The extremely restricted availability of good quality water and the poor quality of the available ground-water in much of the district is the biggest bane of the people of Mewat. The major source of water for human consumption is by harnessing groundwater in the district (IRRAD and Aide et Action, Undated). However, the quality of groundwater in most of the district is very poor and brackish due to its high mineral content. Leave aside human consumption, this water is not even fit for agricultural use (Khan, 2007). Potable water is found underground mostly in the fall of the Aravalli foothills, but even this water has a high nitrate and fluoride content and, as such, is harmful for human consumption. This source of water is fast depleting due to intensive harnessing to meet the water needs of the people in different parts of the district. Efforts have been made to improve the quality of this water by preventing the runoff of rain water from the hills to recharge the ground-water (Sharma et al., undated). However, even this supply becomes erratic owing to the uncertainty of electricity supply, especially in summer and due to poor maintenance of pipes carrying water to distant villages. These pipes were initially laid sometime in the 1960s. With the falling water table in the villages situated along the foothills, there is growing resistance from the people of these villages to letting their water be supplied to distant villages and incidents of piped supply being disrupted by them are not infrequent.

The better-off people in the villages also manage their water needs by purchasing tanker water and storing it in underground water tanks. Apart from public water supply and tanker water, the other sources of drinking water in the district are open wells, bore-wells/tube-wells, and public and private hand-pumps (IRRAD and Aide et Action, undated).

It is important to underline here the social and economic impact of water scarcity on the lives of the people. The struggle for water brings into sharp focus the power relations between the people in rural Mewat, and it is the powerful who seem to enjoy the first right to water. In most villages the piped supply invariably reaches only the houses of the better-off and dominant sections of the people. The piped supply first either goes to the houses of the powerful sections of people in the villages or else the dominant households cut off supply to the poorer households in order to garner a larger share of water. As to the rest, they have to make do with water from the common open village wells which are fed by public water supply, and the poorer households have to fetch water from there. Needless to say, the burden of this drudgery falls on the women of the household. In summer, when piped water supply becomes erratic, the problem of arranging for water reaches crisis proportions with entire families, including children, having to pitch in to carry water from long distances, thereby foregoing the daily wage of at least one or two earning members of the family. Water obtained with such labour is strictly rationed for cooking and drinking purposes, giving a go by to the needs of maintaining personal hygiene and sanitation. The only saving grace is that in Mewat no one is denied access to common water sources on the basis of caste, creed, or religion; the only inequity in here lies in the household's economic capacity.

Status of Agriculture in Mewat

In a district that is over 95 per cent rural with an overwhelming proportion of its people dependent on agriculture and allied activities for sustenance, the role of agriculture in the overall development of the district cannot be overemphasized. The productivity of farms and farm animals in Mewat is very low compared to the otherwise agriculturally prosperous state of

Haryana. Besides, the general neglect of agriculture by the governments in India has an especially deleterious impact on the agricultural economy of backward regions like Mewat.

In Mewat, agriculture is largely rain-fed and practised on small and marginal farms. In most parts of the district a single crop is grown in the year, and only a prospect of a second crop if the rains have been good. Even though nearly 70 per cent of the cultivated area is irrigated, only about 30-35 per cent of the area is economically irrigable, and of that also only 10-15 per cent is irrigated with good quality water (Chauhan et al., undated).

The soil quality of much of the district is very poor with a high salt content, and as such is not very conducive for agriculture (Khan, 2007). Rubbing in the salt, during the green revolution period many farmers shifted to high-yielding varieties of mustard and wheat (Chauhan et al., undated) which require substantial amounts of water, fertilizers, and pesticides, resources for which are wanting with a majority of the small and marginal peasants in the district, but even if they are employed, there are no commensurate returns given the adverse agro-climatic conditions of the district.

Buffaloes and goats form the base of animal husbandry here. However, these are of a local breed and their productivity is poor (Chauhan et al., undated).

Within Mewat almost all the villages are linked by pucca (metalled) roads to the major towns in the district. There are six regulated markets and sub-yards in the district where farmers can sell their produce. However, the transport system in the district is poorly developed and in the absence of any rail link, notwithstanding close physical proximity to cities like Gurgaon, Alwar, and the national capital, Delhi, the farmers have difficulty in accessing the markets of these cities (Chauhan, D.R., undated). Even though there are extension services of the agriculture and the animal husbandry departments in the district along with one KVK (Krishi Vigyan Kendra, the Agriculture Science Centre) of the Chaudhary Charan Singh Haryana Agricultural University, these have been of little help in increasing the productivity and the incomes of the farmers.

Table 4 below shows the proportions of operational landholding by size. It is clear from the distribution of landholdings

Table 4: Proportion of Landholdings by Size

Large (>10 acres)			*Medium(5-10 acres)*			*Small (2-5 acres)*			*Marginal (<2 acres)*			*Landless HH*
No. of hold.	%	*Area (ha)*	*No. of hold.*	%	*Area (ha)*	*No. of hold.*	%	*Area (ha)*	*No. of hold.*	%	*Area (ha)*	*No. of HH*
4,742	2.4	25,971	7,209	7.5	30,068	48,773	21.8	78,576	52,654	68.2	32,135	25,464

Source: Chauhan et al., undated.

Note: These figures include the figures for Hatin block which became part of a new district, Palwal, which was created subsequently.

that overwhelming majority (90 per cent) of farmers in Mewat are small and marginal, and there is a sizable number of landless households. This, along with the other factors mentioned above, has important consequences for the material well-being of the people of the area and impacts their existential needs.

Access to land, as elsewhere in India, means power and social status. It is the powerful who have greater, if not exclusive, access to societal and public resources. We have already seen above how the rich and the dominant sections of people in Mewat have control over water. Similarly, institutional credit is also accessible to the larger landholders in the region. Most of the small and marginal farmers have to rely on the urban trading class for credit to invest in agriculture. As these are small farmers, they have limited holding capacity and are forced to sell whatever marketable surplus produce they have immediately after the harvest, i.e. when the prices are the lowest, and that too invariably to the traders to whom they are indebted. Similarly, even with dairy farming, the smaller farmers have to avail of loans from private moneylenders, meaning thereby that they have to sell their milk to these traders in order to repay the loans and are therefore unable to realize the best price for their produce.

As there is no rail link in the district, this means that there is no means of rapidly transporting their produce, and at an economical cost, to the larger cities in the adjoining districts where they can realize a higher price for it (Chauhan et al., undated). The net result of all this is that for an overwhelming number of people in the district, life is a ceaseless, daily struggle to make two ends meet and in which the first priority is eking out their daily bread, with health and education being pushed down the scale. The dismal state of agriculture in the district means that landless households are able to obtain less work within the district and invariably have to go elsewhere in search of it.

Status of Education in Mewat

Educational development of a people is an important parameter of their overall development. Apart from the social, political, and cultural dimensions, education has increasingly acquired an economic dimension because it is recognized that it leads to the formation of human capital and thereby the development of society (Upadhyay, 2007). Knowledge gained through education can be leveraged to transform oneself and society as a whole. However, it would be exceptional if educational development were to occur irrespective of development in the economic and other social spheres of life, and this is unsurprisingly true of Mewat.

Fig. 1: Comparison of the Literacy Levels of Mewat with Those of Haryana

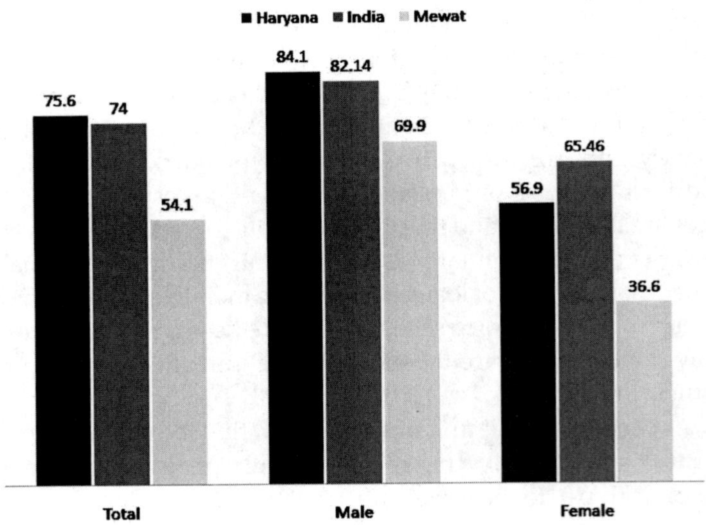

Source: GOI, (2013), *Census of India*, 2013a and 2013b.

Mewat is considerably backward in literacy levels compared to other districts of Haryana and those of the adjoining states of Rajasthan and Uttar Pradesh. Fig. 1 provides a comparison of the levels of literacy in Mewat with those of India as a whole and Haryana in accordance with the findings of the 2011 census (GOI 2013, *Census of India* 2013a, *Census of India* 2013b).

Even though there is an increase in the literacy figures since the 2001 Census, the quality of education leaves much to be desired. Conversations with people of the district reveal that there is a general state of disinterestedness on the part of the government to improve the quality of schools in Mewat. The overall condition of the infrastructure of the schools of Mewat is dismal. The buildings are either in need for major repairs or there the classrooms lack furniture for the students. Essential facilities such as drinking water and toilets are invariably missing and the teacher-student ratio in all the blocks can vary from anywhere between 50:1 to 80:1 (IRRAD and Aide et Action, undated).

However, the lack of infrastructure in the schools is only one of the stumbling blocks in improving the educational standards of Mewat. There are far more formidable reasons that are rooted in the real-life conditions of the people of Mewat. Education has been enshrined as a fundamental right in the Constitution with the passage of the 'Right to Education Act' in 2010. However, given the perfunctory nature in which the right to education is implemented in India, de facto it translates into one-sided emphasis on primary education; as regards higher levels of education, neither is the government interested nor do the real-life conditions of the poor people permit them this liberty, especially where the more existential needs of life take priority. Data shows that the schools of Mewat register a precipitous fall in enrolment rates after primary school (Tables 5 and 6). There is a sharp decrease in the number of medium, higher secondary, and senior secondary schools compared to primary schools, as also in the enrolment rates to the higher standards. Whereas primary schools are 22 times larger in number than senior secondary schools, the ratio of enrolment in the primary schools to that in the senior secondary is 29: 1.

Table 5: Detail of Government Schools in Mewat District

Category of School	*Boys*	*Girls*	*Total*
Primary school	444	87	**531**
Middle school	218	54	**272**
High school	39	05	**44**
Sr. Secondary school	20	04	**24**
New Model school			**06**
Total	**721**	**150**	**871**

Source: Mewat Development Agency.
Note: This figure includes the statistics for Hatin block of Palwal district as that also falls under the jurisdiction of the MDA.

Table 6: Total Enrolment and the Gender Ratio in Mewat District (Class I to 12)

Class	*Boys*	*Girls*	*Boys : Girls*	*Total*
Government Schools				
I to 5	74,555	61,605	1.2:1	1,36,160
6 to 8	18,965	8,933	2.12:1	27,898
9 to 10	5,320	2,126	2.5:1	7,446
11 to 12	3,569	1,118	3.2:1	4,687
Total	**1,02,409**	**73,782**	**1.4:1**	**1,76,191**

Source: Mewat Development Agency.
Note: This figure includes the statistics for Hatin block of Palwal district as that also comes under the jurisdiction of the MDA.

It is very evident from Table 5 that with regard to enrolment in schools, the ratio of boys is much greater than that for girls, with this gap progressively increasing in favour of boys in higher classes.

An additional issue is that of the availability of qualified teachers in the region. It is not uncommon to find that many of the teachers in the villages of Mewat have been posted from other districts of Haryana. In a study conducted by the Institute of Rural Research and Development (IRRAD) in 20 villages of Mewat spread across all the blocks of the district, it was found that of the 20 teachers interviewed, only three, were postgraduates, five were graduates and 60 per cent of the teachers had just passed the twelfth standard (IRRAD and Aide et Action, undated). Another problem is that the proportion of female teachers is very low, which creates additional problems in the cultural milieu of Mewat which is heavily influenced by what can be described as 'religious obscurantism'.

Indeed, it is true that there are important cultural barriers to the rapid spread of education in Mewat. As an activist of one NGO, Mewat Social and Educational Development Society, put it, that the attitude to educating children was till very recently: *'Thoda Padha Kaam Se Gaya, Jyada Padha Gaon Se Gaya'* (even a semi-educated person shirks physical labour, while a well read one just leaves the village) (Singh, C.P., 2008). These attitudes have changed considerably over the past decade or so and people now want their children to be educated. However, the fact remains that modern education has done very little to advance the agricultural way of life of the Meos. Besides, in the absence of avenues for employment, modern education has not brought the expected dividends for the younger generation. School pass-outs playing cards is a common sight in the villages of Mewat. People even complained that educated youth are no longer interested in the back-breaking agricultural work. These factors do make the rapid spread of literacy into a Catch-22 situation.

There are about 215 madrasas (Muslim religious schools) in the district which attract a considerable number of pupils. They have separate rooms for girls and boys (Planning Commission, 2005). As an empirical fact, the religion-centric view of education may be undeniable; the point however is how do we understand these perceptions?

Government Action to Improve Literacy

According to the budget allocations of the Mewat Development Authority for different sectors for the years 2009-10 and 2010-11, development of educational institutions has been one of the clear priorities with education garnering a lion's share of the developmental funds at 23 and 59.12 per cent respectively for the two years.

As is true of the rest of India, education in Mewat is also of two kinds: one for the rich and the other for the poor. This is effected not only through separate private schools for the better off but finds reflection even within the government sector. The government of Haryana in collaboration with the Mewat Development Agency started two English-medium co-educational schools at Nuh and Ferozpur Jirkha in 1985-6 with the express 'objective of promoting quality education as a key to prosperity in a distinct ethnic and socio-cultural tract' (Mewat Development Agency, 2011c) under the auspices of the Mewat Model Schools Society. Subsequently, one Model School was established in each block of the district. Table 7 sets out the fee structure of these schools, and this needs to be examined in light of the fact that over 90 per cent of the peasant households in this overwhelmingly rural district are the small and marginal, with incomes that make daily sustenance a challenge. Besides these, a significant proportion of the population in the district comprises landless agricultural labour. Excluding the registration fee, the caution money, and the monthly expenditure on conveyance, the monthly expenditure for a single student of the primary section in these Model Schools is Rs. 306; adding a minimum of Rs. 200 per month for conveyance, the expenditure on just one child will be nearly equal to the then rural poverty line for Haryana, which was Rs. 529.40 per month and exceeded two-third of the urban poverty line of Rs. 626.41 per month (Planning Commission, 2011). These realities mean that, given their fee structure and the medium of instruction, the Model Schools are certainly not meant for the general population of the district.

Table 7: Fee Structure of Mewat Model Schools

Sr. No.	*Fee Head*	*Class*	*Amount (Rs)*
1.	Registration	Nur. to V	150.00
		VI to X	200.00
		XI to XII	250.00
2.	Caution money once at the time of admission	Nur. to V	150.00
		VI to X	200.00
		XI to XII	250.00
3.	Annual charges	Nur to KG	400.00
		I to V	700.00
		VI to X	900.00
		XI & XII	1050.00
4.	Exams charges per annum	Nur. to V	150.00
		VI to X	200.00
		XI to XII	250.00
5.	Monthly tuition fees	Nur. to KG	200.00
		I to V	250.00
		VI to X	300.00
		XI & XII	525.00
6.	Computer fees	Nur. & KG	Exempted
		Ist to 5th	35.00
		6th to 10th	40.00
		10+I & II	75.00
7.	Conveyance fees	Upto 5 KM	200.00 PM
		5 to 10 KM	300.00 PM
		Above 10 KM	400.00 PM

Source: Mewat Development Agency, Mewat Model Schools Society, Nuh.

Besides the 'Model Schools', the MDA also runs six Kasturba Gandhi Balika Vidyalyas, which are residential schools for girls of the scheduled and backward castes, and those from the minority community and below poverty line families (BPL). According to the details available at the Mewat Development Agency website, there are a number of government ITIs (industrial training institutes) and polytechnics in the district; Mewat Development Authority even runs an 'Institute of Hospitality Management' at Nuh offering diploma courses in 'Food production' and 'Food & Beverage Service' (Mewat Development Agency, 2011 c), even though there is no hospitality industry worth a name in the district. Whatever be the rationale behind such investments in education, they are certainly not geared to meet the present needs of the people, nor is the development of Mewat taking place in a way that can harness the present education facilities to facilitate development of the region. For example, there could certainly be at least one agricultural college in this predominantly rural and agricultural district. A new government medical college has recently opened in Nuh block but it remains to be seen as to what avenues it will provide to local students to become doctors and the degree to which those benefiting will be willing to serve the people of their district.

The madrasas (religious seminaries)/maktabs have traditionally been an important substitute for school education in Mewat, especially in relation to women's education. These schools have been relatively untouched by the modern developments in Islamic theology. Even until a decade ago the *nisab* (syllabus) of most of these madrasas was in conformity with *dars-i-nizami*, prepared way back in the time of Mughal Emperor Aurangzeb. The widely held perception of the Meos was that their children would not in any case get jobs and needed to look after family farms and therefore modern education held little promise for them. That was why knowledge of *din* (religion) was thought to be sufficient. This perception has loosened only in the past decade or so, but still holds largely true for girls (Sikand, 1995).

Sanitation in Mewat

Sanitary conditions in Mewat are acutely wanting. According to the DLHS – 3 survey, a total of 16.2 per cent households in Mewat had a toilet facility, while in the rural areas this figure dropped to 12.2 per cent. According to one government survey, the proportion of Hindus and Muslims who defecate in the open is around 91.31 and 86.30 per cent respectively, while the Hindu and Muslim settlements without any drainage facility are 27.62 per cent and 41.45 per cent respectively (Institute of Human Development, 2008).

It need hardly be emphasized that this has important consequences for the health of the people. The Total Sanitation Campaign has proved to be a non-starter in Mewat (Institute of Human Development, 2008); neither is there any apparent emphasis on the part of the district health administration to achieve the targets set out for the campaign. The few sanitary latrines that had been built in some villages with the help of an NGO, IRRAD (Institute of Rural Research and Development), have also fallen into disuse due to a scarcity of water.

Nutritional Status in Mewat

For its low level of social and economic development with poor health indicators, it is quite surprising that there have been no large-scale surveys undertaken by the government to estimate the magnitude of malnutrition in Mewat. However, given the overall scenario, malnutrition is a very serious problem, particularly among women and children.

With over two-thirds of the rural population beset with a low standard of living, qround 50 per cent of the girls being married before the age of 18 years (GOI, 2007-8), early age of pregnancy, and large family size, problems like anaemia and wasting are rampant among women. Only about 7.6 per cent of the babies are breastfed within an hour of birth (GOI, 2007-8). A low level of immunization and poor sanitation are very likely to ensure a regular cycle of malnutrition and infections feeding on each other to result in a higher than average proportion of wasting and stunting among children.

Status of Women in Mewat

Any discussion on the backwardness of Mewat cannot be complete without discussing the status of women in Mewat. The general economic and educational backwardness of a place has consequences for its cultural development and also its societal values. Mewat's socio-economic status has not surpisingly weighed heavy on the status of its women too.

Although women in the district have a considerable productive role in the agricultural and dairy farms besides home responsibilities such as fetching water, firewood, washing clothes, cooking, bearing the burden of repeated pregnancies, and rearing the children, their recognition in the villages is almost exclusively on account of their reproductive role. They have little say in household decisions, or even in control over their fertility and virtually no say in public life (IRRAD, 2010). The average age of marriage of women in the area is just 13 years. They bear their first child by the age of 14 or 15 years, and on an average a Meo woman has 18 pregnancies (Singh, C.P., 2008).

The social and economic disempowerment of women is reflected in their abysmally low share in work participation rates. The work participation rate among Hindu and the Muslim women is 6.72 and 5.61 per cent respectively. By comparison, the work participation rate among Hindu and Muslim males is 43.36 and 38.04 per cent respectively (Institute of Human Development, 2008).

In addition to the conservative and feudal value system of the people in the district, the hardships of daily life, be it on account of scarcity of water or lack of education only serves to enslave women not just physically but also mentally. In the IRRAD study on gender equity in the district, in response to the question whether men are superior to women, 71 per cent women and 76 per cent men replied in affirmative (Institute of Human Development, 2008).

An abhorrent attitude towards women is particularly borne out by the reported practice by families of buying women from other parts of India such as Assam, West Bengal, Bihar, and Orissa to work as sex slaves for men in the family or for marriage (Joshi, 2003). This practice of women trafficking is known to extend well beyond Mewat to other areas of Haryana (in the districts dominated by Jat caste), areas of Punjab, and Western UP tool.

Even though the practice is far too often ascribed to the low sex ratio of the state, rather than understanding the roots of the problem and remedying them, this may only be a convenient way of explaining it away. Indeed, if a low sex ratio is such a powerful driving force then the relative social position of women in Haryana should have been strengthened and practices such as dowry should have declined and women should have had a greater say in choosing their husbands, but such a scenario remains as distant as ever.

Even though the practice of accepting dowry is not permitted in Islam, it is widely prevalent among Meos; either because of their Hindu ancestry or because of the influence of the Hindu population surrounding their villages (*Tribune*, 2004).

Nature of Politics in the District

In the kind of electoral politics that has come to prevail in India, welfare of the people has become ephemeral to the life and blood of politics. Money, muscle power, and tools to manipulate public opinion increasingly determine the fortune of the political parties and political leaders. Under these circumstances, an illiterate, impoverished, conservative, and politically immobilized public that asks few questions regarding the conditions of its existence can only be regarded as a coveted political base by the political parties. The people of Mewat easily conform to all these characteristics.

Another factor that is seldom acknowledged in official circles or even in academic discourse is that the Meos are neglected because they are a minority and have traditionally been looked upon with suspicion and contempt by the establishment. The fact of Mewat being a Muslim-dominated area was cited by a couple of people, though in a guarded way, as being an important reason for its backwardness. If the findings of the Sachar Committee on the 'Social, Economic and Educational Status of the Muslim Community of India' (GOI, 2006) are anything to go by, then such a feeling need not be considered to be ill-founded as is discussed later in the chapter.

There are no mass youth or women's or peasants' organizations even of the mainstream political parties, that are willing to take up and build struggles on the multifarious issues of the people in Mewat. Local politics in the villages is totally controlled by the landed élite.

Table 8: Average Population Per CHC, PHC, Sub-Centre, and Status of Sub-Centre Building

CHC	*Avg. popul. under each CHC*	*No. of PHCs under the CHC*	*Avg. popul under each PHC*	*No. of sub-centres under the CHC*	*Avg. popul per sub-centre*	*Status of sub-centre building*				*Status of govt. bldg.*	
						Government		*Private*	*Working in PHC*	*Good*	*Bad*
						Funct-ioning	*Non-Funct-ional*				
1. Nuh	4,24,381	5	1,13,517	32	13,254	6	7	15	4	6	7
2. Punhana	2,32,260	4	58,065	27	10,971	6	11	7	3	6	11
3. F.P. Jhirka	2,79,112	4	69,778	25	10,988	5	8	8	4	5	8
Total	-	13	-	84		17	26	30	11	17	26

Source: Compiled from figures provided in Civil Surgeon Mewat, 2010. (Civil Surgeon Mewat, 2010: District Action Plan, Mewat 2010-11.)

Table 9: Number of Health Institutions Available/Required/Sanctioned as per the Population Norm

Recommended population norm for health institutions	*Required no. of health institutions in Mewat as per 2001 population norm*	*Available no. of health institutions*			*New health institutions*		*Total of available + sanctioned + sanction awaited*
		Government Building	*Non-government buildings*	*Total*	*New sanctioned*	*Sanction awaited*	
1 Sub-centre per 5,000 population	190	43	41	84 (44.2)	54	Nil	138 (72.6)
1 PHC per 30,000 population	30	8	5	13 (43.4)	7	3	23 (76.7)
1 CHC per 1 lakh population	8	3	–	3 (37.5)	-	3	6 (75)

Source: Based on the information provided by the office of the Civil Surgeon, Mewat. Note: Figures in parenthesis are the proportions of total requirement in accordance with the norms.

Health Infrastructure and Manpower

The health infrastructure of Mewat is still in its infancy compared with the rest of Haryana state. It lacks both in the required number of health institutions warranted by the population norms, as also the quality of care provided by the available institutions. The private health set-up conforming to the standards of modern health care is non-existent in the district.

Tables 8 and 9 show the acute deficiency of health infrastructure in Mewat. The actual deficiency of infrastructure is much greater than is reflected in these tables because many of the facilities are either functioning in rented structures, which is a constraint on making the full complement of services available, or more than one health institution is functioning from a single premise. Inter-alia health institutions that ought to have had a much wider reach become restricted in access besides there is a duplication of services and inefficient functioning.

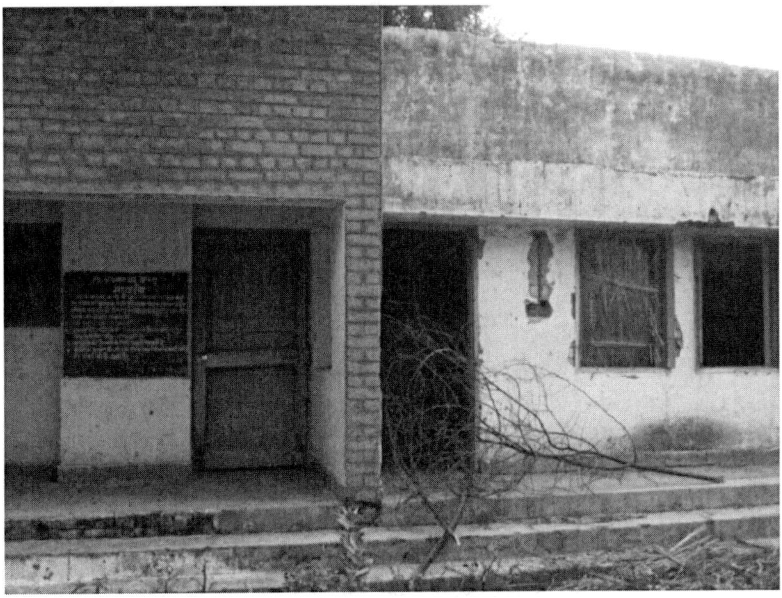

Fig. 2a: State of disrepair at sub-centre Nawli, under PHC F.P. Jhirka

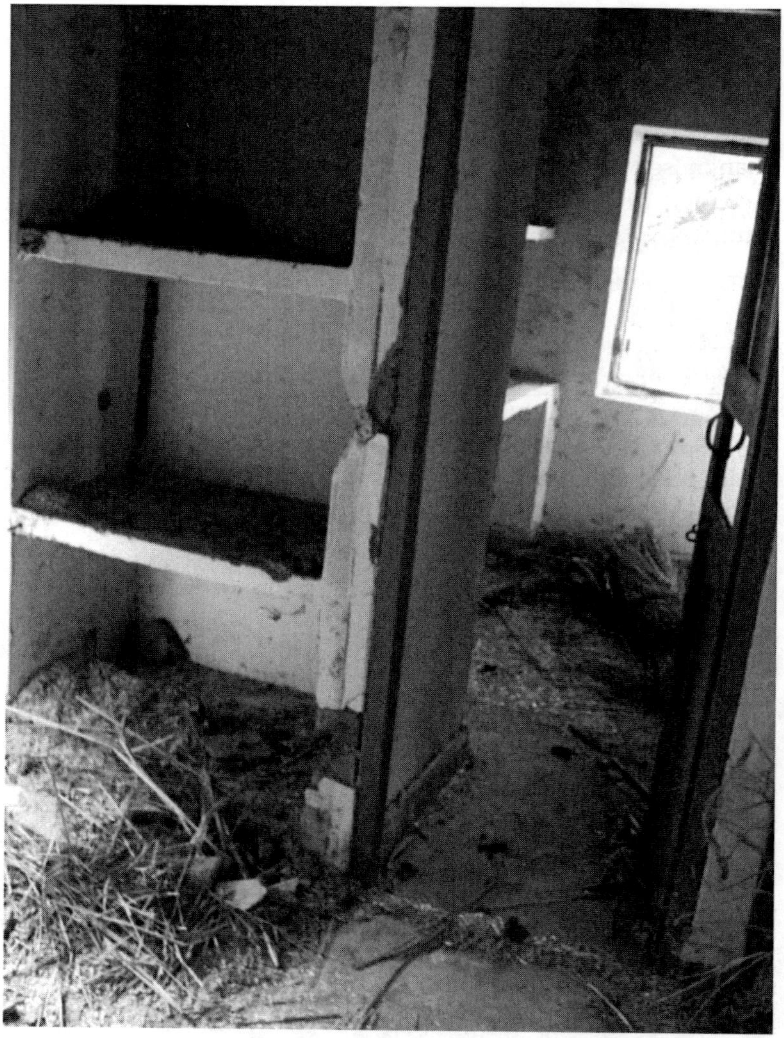

Fig. 2b: Interiors of sub-centre at Nawli used perhaps for storing farm produce

The utter state of disrepair of some of the buildings (Figs. 2a and 2b) gives an impression that their present state could have come about only under conditions of disuse and total neglect. Figs.

2a and 2b show the condition of the sub-centre at Nawli under PHC Firozpur Jhirka. It is difficult to believe that this building was rebuilt only in 1991. As is clear from Table 8, there are more sub-centres located in government buildings that are non-functional than those that are functional.

Table 10 gives the overall medical and paramedical manpower situation in the district as in 2010.

Table 10: Overall Health Manpower Situation in District Mewat, District Action Plan 2010-11

Designation	*Sanctioned*	*Regular Filled*	*Regular Vacant Posts*
Civil surgeon	1	1	0
Programme officer	7	4	03 (42.86)
Senior medical officer	4	1	03 (75.00)
Medical officers	70	60	10 (14.30)
Dental surgeon	17	13	04 (23.53)
Staff nurse	45	9	36 (80.00)
Lab. tech.	23	1	22 (95.65)
Radiographer	6	6	0
MPHW (M)	84	11	73 (86.90)
MPHW (F)	84	36	48 (57.14)
MPHS (M)	16	9	07 (43.75)
MPHS (F)	18	7	11 (61.11)
Opthal. asstt.	4	1	03 (75.00)
Pharmacist	18	6	12 (66.66)
Class IV	73	37	36 (49.31)
Total	471	201	270

Source: Civil Surgeon Mewat, 2010.
Note: MPHW = Multi Purpose Health Worker; MPHS = Multi Purpose Health Supervisor. SMI* (not known). Note: The figures in parenthesis are vacancies as a proportion of sanctioned posts.

Infrastructure and Functioning of the District Hospital

The Al-Afia general hospital at Mandi Kheda can easily be counted as one of the most imposing buildings in the entire district (Fig. 3). Spread over an area of 17 acres, this campus has a hospital building and residential quarters for doctors and employees along with a great deal of open space.

Fig. 3: Al-Afia General Hospital at Mandi Kheda, Mewat

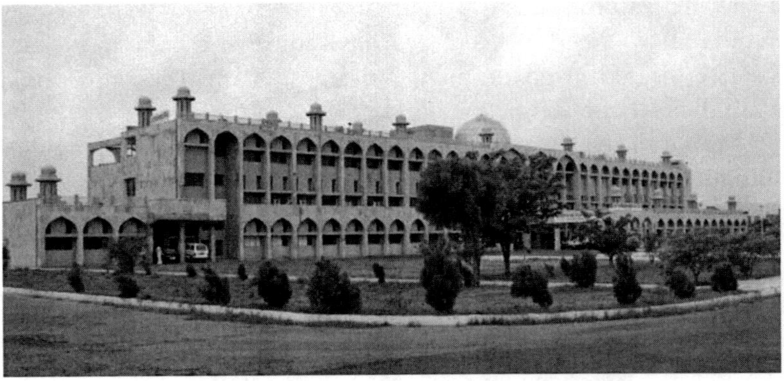

The district hospital has a total of 50 inpatient beds as against the suggested norm of 200 beds at a district hospital for a population of 10,000 (Planning Commission, 2011). There are OPD services for different disciplines, a labour room, and an operation theatre. However, in the absence of specialist doctors such as a gynaecologist and obstetrician, a general surgeon, a ENT surgeon, etc. the OPDs are managed by the internists or general duty medical officers. At the time of the study, two paediatricians, two ophthalmologists, two orthopaedic surgeons (one on contract basis), two physicians, and one dermatologist were available at the hospital.

In the absence of an anaesthetist, only some minor surgeries were performed under loco-regional anaesthesia, e.g. hernia and cataract. The emergency services are capable of handling simple medical emergencies, simple fractures, provision of first aid for severe trauma cases and clean lacerated wounds, etc. Complicated cases are all referred to Gurgaon or the patients may go to Delhi or Alwar. Centralized ambulance services are available to ferry the patients. Owing to the non-availability of a gynaecologist and obstetrician, the hospital is not equipped to handle any obstetrical emergencies. Only normal deliveries are conducted at the hospital 24 X 7, by the staff nurses.

The hospital has one laboratory with one lab technician that undertakes only limited haematological, urine and stool investigations. There are two X-ray machines for taking simple radiographs; no special radiographs are taken. There is no blood bank facility; however a blood-storage facility is available.

Infrastructural Facilities at the CHCs

All the CHCs provide only routine OPD services and provide 24 hour delivery services for uncomplicated cases. Under the circumstances, none of the CHCs are serving as FRUs (First Referral Units) to strengthen the peripheral health services and to provide specialist care closest to the people.

What Ails the Health of the People in Mewat: Perceptions of Health and other Government Functionaries (C)

An attempt was made during the course of this study to understand how the health and other important government functionaries conceptualized the problems of the people and contrast their perceptions with how the people themselves articulated their needs. This was considered necessary to understand the capacity of the health services to effectively deal with the felt and epidemiologically determined health needs of the people.

Perceptions of Doctors

The different doctors interviewed during the course of the study were asked what they thought were the measures that needed to be taken for the development of Mewat and improvement of the health of the people, in their order of significance. The following issues were cited by the doctors, including the Civil Surgeon, in the order of their significance:

1. Improving literacy and avenues for education.
2. Large family size.
3. Improving the health infrastructure.
4. Strong religious beliefs were identified as an important obstacle for adoption of progressive steps such as family planning, women's education, and improvement in women's health.
5. Deficiency of water.
6. Some doctors also spoke of improving the living and working conditions of doctors and facilities for them such as education of their children, to motivate more doctors to be wiling to work in Mewat.

The Civil Surgeon, Dr. K.S. Rao, identified the deficiency of water as an important impediment in the development of the region; others mentioned it only as an afterthought or agreed to such a need when it was suggested. Outdated religious beliefs were cited as an important obstacle for the development of the region, e.g. this was the main reason for the large size of the families, which led to a deficiency of resources; this was also considered to be an obstacle to modern education, especially the education of women, which led to all kinds of social taboos.

None of the respondents mentioned the need to take measures to modernize agriculture in the region, improving the transport facilities there, the need to adopt other measures for the economic well-being of the district such as setting up industries or laying of railway lines across the district.

The response of the former Civil Surgeon of the district, Dr. H.S. Randhawa, was along similar lines and was cited in one of the studies by Helpage India. He is quoted as saying: 'a major cause of the diseases the Meo people suffer from is the lack of awareness, lack of education, lack of balanced diet and the resulting low haemoglobin content' (Singh, C.P., 2008).

Perceptions of the MPHWs and ASHAs

The responses of the MPHWs (Multipurpose Health Workers) and the ASHAs (Accredited Social Health Activists) with respect to having an understanding of the socio-economic issues relating to health did not go beyond parroting the official bylines, e.g. if the deliveries are done at home then there is danger to the life of the mother and the baby, and therefore there is a need to motivate women to opt for institutional deliveries. The ASHA workers were not even aware of NRHM; their only refrain being institutional deliveries and immunization. The MPHWs, though they were aware of NRHM, were dismal in their conceptualization of how socio-economic issues impact on health. Their response to what was required to be done to improve the condition of health of the people was limited to advocacy of institutional deliveries, immunization, consumption of green leafy vegetables, breastfeeding, and the like.

Perceptions of School Teachers

A teacher is looked upon as a person of importance and commands considerable respect, especially in a rural setting. They can be expected to have some realistic understanding of the issues in the daily lives of the people.

The teachers interviewed during this study were all teaching at the primary and middle schools at Uleta village. In order to simplify matters, no questions were posed to them regarding the health problems of the people in the area. They were only asked to express their opinion on the principal reasons for the lack of development in the district. It is important to mention here that of the five teachers present, three were Hindu and two were Meo Muslims; of the three Hindu teachers, two were from outside the district and had been posted in the school at Uleta for over two years. Even as the conversation began, the two Meo teachers left for the mosque to offer Friday afternoon prayers; this perhaps facilitated a freer expression of opinion by the others.

Rather than expressing their considered opinions on the problems of underdevelopment in the area by the two teachers who were from outside the district, vociferously began complaining about the people themselves. Their first refrain was that:

> The people here do not realize the importance of education. They are not bothered whether having left the home their child has gone to school or not; they think that education takes place only in schools and as soon as the child is back from school they will send her/him to the forest to fetch some wood or to the fields to cut *bathua* (white goosefoot) as this is the season for that. Parents do not consider it important to sit with their children at home and ensure that they study.

Their further concern was:

> They do not consider the school to be their own; a mandir. It ought to be equally respected as their mosque, but they have already stolen all the window bars from the new classrooms that were built for the middle section ... they come and defecate in the classrooms.

The high crime rate was the other major problem of the district according to these teachers. They maintained that 'the people here are very clever and can befool anyone easily'. They went on to describe the type of crimes being committed in the district, as if they were policemen contemptuously lamenting the criminal nature of the people. The 'people', in their arguments, was underpinned by an unspoken reference to the Meos.

The third, but no less important problem they raised was that of religious fundamentalism coupled with the large number of children in families. People, it was said, gave greater importance to the instructions of the *maulvi* in the mosque than to what was taught in school. According to them, the local Hindus said that the 'large number of children among the Muslim families led them also to have more children too so that there would be enough men in the family to ensure protection from Meos in the event of a dispute'.

A semblance of balance was brought to the discussion by the local Hindu teacher who said that the availability of potable water was the biggest problem of Mewat. His perspective was further enriched by the Meo teachers who had returned after the prayers. Speaking about the backwardness of Mewat, one of them said that in many Mewat villages women have to date not even seen a train. This one statement speaks volumes about the level of development or lack of it right in the backyard of the national capital.

People's Perception of Development and Their Felt Needs

The opinions expressed in this section were gathered through informal discussions, in-depth interviews, and through semi-structured interview schedules to people from different strata/ socio-economic categories in Uleta village of Nagina block of the distrct which was being studied.

Household no. 1, head of family (HOF) Mohd. Isa, belonged to the dominant households of the Meo community and was located in the sarpanch's (village headman) locality; household no. 2, HOF, Leela Ram was from a BPL household; and household no. 3, HOF Sampat Ram, from a non-BPL household (the latter two were from the poor Scheduled Caste community); household no. 4, HOF Ram Singh, was from the generally affluent Brahmin upper caste community of the village; household no. 5, HOF Husain Shah and household no. 6, HOF Roshan were from a BPL non-Meo Muslim households. The interviews with these households provided different perspectives and insights into the life of the people in the village, as also those of the people in the area in general. Depending upon their socio-economic conditions, they had different demands/ expectations from the government.

Among all the questions the respondents in each of the households were asked what development measures would they like the government to take in the order of priority which they thought would bring about a fundamental change in their lives. The answers to the question of different households varied depending upon their socio-economic background. It was striking that the people's priorities were in stark contrast to the way development is viewed by government functionaries. These opinions have an important bearing even on the manner in which improvement in the health of the people ought to be brought about.

Cutting across the socio-economic strata, a long-term solution to the problem of water scarcity in the area was the first demand of all the households. However, the perceptions regarding the kind of solution varied between the more affluent and the BPL households. For the more affluent households (households 1 and 4), the demand was for a viable solution to meet the irrigation needs of the farmers to enable a more remunerative agriculture in the region. These households had comparatively large landholdings and irrigation of their lands would have a direct impact on increasing their prosperity.

In contrast to the affluent households, for the BPL households (households 5 and 6) and the non-BPL Dalit household (household 3), the first priority was water for household use because, unlike the richer households, they neither had household piped water supply nor could they afford to purchase water easily in the summer months when the scarcity was most acute. Scarcity of drinking water had a very direct impact on their economic well-being, especially during summer months, as a sizable part of the family's day was spent on fetching water from nearby villages, causing at least some of the earning members to forego their daily wages. Once their daily need for water was satisfied, these households wanted water to be available for agricultural use on a sustainable basis as more prosperous agriculture would mean locally available employment opportunities as wage labourers on the farms of the bigger farmers, besides having spinoff benefits for dairy farming and other economic activities. This would obviate the need, at least for a considerable part of the year, for them to go to distant places in search of work, and in consequence spending more on travel as well as having to bear additional living expenses away from home.

The second priority for the more affluent households was a railway line connecting Mewat with the cities of Delhi and Gurgaon, on the one hand, and Alwar on the other. Their take on the issue was that besides facilitating cheaper and quicker transport to the bigger cities, this would enable them to make a larger profit by directly selling their produce such as milk or vegetables in the markets of these cities. A rail link would also facilitate easier access to the job markets of the adjoining cities for the educated youth of these households without them having to move away from their families in Mewat.

While a rail link would facilitate easier and cheaper access to job markets of cities like Delhi, Gurgaon, and Alwar even for the poorer households, yet these households (households 4, 5 and 6) placed the need for a pucca house above the need for a rail link. The present kuccha, dialapidated houses of these families afforded them less protection from the vagaries of the weather and as such a more secure dwelling was a much more pressing need than the distant dream of a rail link.

The third most important need of the more affluent households (households 1 and 4) and household 3 was for some local industry to be developed in Mewat to enable the educated youth of the district to find gainful employment rather than just loiter around as they now did. The poorer households were supportive of the idea but did not articulate this on their own. The wife of Leela Ram, a rickshaw-puller (household 2) seemed much too despondent to have any expectations at all.

It is clearly evident that the more affluent households nurture aspirations for the fulfilment of their needs. Even on as fundamental an issue as water, their orientation is of finding ways of increasing their prosperity. The BPL households, on the other hand, are so far removed from aspirations of a prosperous life; their orientation towards developmental issues is borne out more from of their existential needs than aspirations for a qualitative improvement in their lives. Indeed, households like that of Leela Ram, an old couple from ostracized caste, totally neglected by government agencies and subsisting below the poverty line have virtually nothing to look up to apart from a faint hope of somehow being able to feed themselves. Households such as that of Sampat Ram (household 3) which lie in between, with some agricultural land and just one son who is graduating, is a rather rare thing in Mewat, have shared aspirations with both the more affluent sections of the people as also the poor because they are positioned where a jump towards greater prosperity can still be dreamt. Regarding the poorer sections, having any hope for a decent life remains as distant as ever.

Remarkably none of the households mentioned the need for better educational or health institutions. When this was pointed out, the respondent in household 1, Mohd. Isa said that once there is greater prosperity for the people they will automatically seeek better educational and health services. As regards the poorer households, their priorities are clear: bread and butter issues come first, education and better health is not on their immediate agenda. This does not mean that they are indifferent to the health institutions; rather they wish them to be more responsive to their health needs which is not currently happening, their consistent refrain regarding the health sub-centre in the village was that it provided only delivery services.[2] Also, the grim struggle for their daily bread affords them few opportunities to care for their health, besides the fact that the material conditions imposed by poverty breed a general apathy towards life itself. This was graphically evident from the large scab-covered ulcer on the face of Husain Shah's (household 5) three-year-old granddaughter which had developed simply because the family missed out on taking her to the doctor when the multiple boils had first appeared. The situation is further compounded by the fact that the sub-centre in the village does not even have the gentian violet to apply on the wound, let alone give her the antibiotics.

Apart from providing services for deliveries and immunization of pregnant women and children, the health sub-centre in the village has made less impact on the daily lives of the people in the village. The better off couldn't care less about the services of the centre because they continue to rely primarily on private doctors, or can get the sub-centre workers to visit their homes as and when the need arises. The poor seek more effective remedial services for their day-to-day curative needs from the centre, but that is just not happening. The destitute of the village like Leela Ram's family remain as ephemeral to the government's schemes as ever; the health workers not even caring to enquire about their welfare.

All in all, rather than being the proverbial fish in water, the sub-centre remains like a splendid drop of oil in water as in terms of integrating the health services with the social life of the village. Rather than forming a part of an integrated development strategy, the development of public health services takes place in isolation from other sectors impacting on health, and this greatly undermines their ability to bring about comprehensive development of people's health.

The other informal opinions on the developmental needs in Mewat that were expressed by different people with whom I interacted in the district conformed to one or the other opinions expressed by the households cited above.

Does Dearth of Water Resources and Poor Agriculture Explain Mewat's Backwardness?

Up to now, I have carefully recorded the various parameters of the socio-economic development of Mewat. This is markedly poor compared to the adjoining districts of the state and also the adjoining districts of the neighbouring states of Rajasthan and Uttar Pradesh. In terms of understanding the reasons of Mewat's backwardness, there seems to be a wide divergence between the reasons and developmental needs of Mewat prioritized by government functionaries and the people themselves. This leaves scope to delve deeper into the reasons for Mewat's backwardness.

Some of the important reasons that have been identified above are acute shortage of water both for domestic and agricultural use, low productivity of agriculture and allied activities, lack of physical infrastructure and the conservative religious thinking that is said to lie at the root of numerous social problems such as large family size, low levels of literacy, especially female literacy, poor status of women in the society, cultural backwardness and poverty.

I would prefer here to adhere to the dictum: 'It is the being that decides the consciousness' rather than adopt a 'victim-blaming' approach of blaming the people's 'attitudes' and 'conservatism' for their backwardness. This implies that backward attitudes and thinking can also be effectively combated by bringing about material development of the living conditions which are expected to lead to the birth of a new and forward-looking approach and ways of thinking. Given this, reasons such as scarcity of water affecting economic activity such as productivity in agriculture and allied activities ought to be considered the central reason for Mewat's backwardness. The straightforward hypothesis is that prosperous agriculture brings about economic development, leading to higher demand and development of health and various other societal institutions. However, it would be prudent to test this hypothesis.

In the following passages I have used the comparative analysis of the development indicators of Mewat and other districts faced with similar conditions, as a heuristic device to explain possible reasons for Mewat's backwardness. The two other districts that I have selected are Mahendergarh which adjoins Mewat within Haryana and Jalore in the adjoining state of Rajasthan. Just like Mewat, both Mahendergarh and Jalore are socio-economically very backward, with poor development indicators and an economy that relies as its mainstay on subsistence agriculture and allied activities. All three districts have semi-arid agro-climatic conditions and face an acute shortage of water both for irrigation and human consumption. While Mahendergarh district is slightly better off in terms of average rainfall, the conditions in Jalore are very dry with the district adjoining the great Indian Thar Desert.

Table 11 provides a comparison of the development indicators of the three districts. It can be seen that although all three districts are beset with a severe water crisis their development indicators indicate a considerable variance. In fact, Jalore's water crisis is much severer than Mewat's as it is an extension of the Thar desert. Though by no means impressive, Jalore's indices are much better than Mewat's. Apart from the proportion of people with a low standard of living index, which is higher for Jalore, Jalore has maternal and child health indicators that are considerably better than Mewat's. Many of the household indicators, including supply of piped drinking water, are much better for Jalore. The much better developed health infrastructure of Jalore is noteworthy compared to Mewat's and even that of Mahendergarh in terms of the population norms for peripheral health services. Jalore's better health infrastructure and maternal and child health indicators have been possible despite its agricultural productivity which is much poorer given its desert conditions.

Table 11: Comparison of Key Indicators of Districts Mewat, Mahendergarh and Jalore

Indicator	*Mewat*	*Mahendergarh*	*Jalore*
Female literacy rate (7 years and above) – 2001 Census	24.26%	54.08%	27.5%
Male literacy rate (7 years and above) – 2001 Census	61.55%	84.72%	65.1%
Total population – 2001 Census	9,93,000	8,13,000	14,48,940
Percentage of urban population	7.07%	13.49%	7.6%
Health Infrastructure*			
No. of secondary care level hospitals	1	1	3
CHC	3	3	8
PHC	13	57	
Sub-Centre	84	100 (40 with delivery huts)	358
AYUSH facilities	1	24	71
Family welfare centres	2	8	-
Private hospitals	12 (a)	-	15
DLHS 3 Data			
Total literate population (Age 7+) %	53.6	75.4	51.5
Hhs having electricity connection %	78.8	89.9	58.2
Hhs having access to toilet facility %	16.2	37.0	11.8
Hhs having piped drinking water %	35.1	78.8	65.6
Hhs using LPG for cooking %	4.5	15.2	10.0
Hhs living in a pucca house %	34.6	51.7	29.2
Hhs having BPL card %	24.5	16.4	21.6
Hh owning agricultural land %	53.7	58.9	64.5
Hhs having a television %	21.4	53.0	24.0
Hhs owning a motorized vehicle %	21.2	24.6	15.2

Standard of Living Index (%)						
Low	64.0	–	40.2	37.3	74.7	70.1
Medium	24.1	–	32.7	40.8	15.2	19.9
High	11.9	–	27.1	22.1	10.1	10.1
Mothers who had 3 antenatal care visits during last pregnancy (%).	16.4	-	54.2	31.9	30.2	20.8
Institutional births (%)	14.8	-	56.8	29.4	35.1	16.4
Children (12-23 mths.) fully immunized (%).	12.2	-	63.0	50.6	51	14.4
Children with diarrhoea in last 2 weeks who received ORS (%).	7.6	-	39.9	20.8	19.0	17.1
Children who had check-up within 24 hrs after delivery, based on last delivery (%)	32.4	-	53.3	-	34.8	-
Children breast-fed within 1 hr of birth (%)	7.6	-	21.1	-	45.1	-

Availability of Water**			
Total irrigated area	88.00%(b)	79.00% (c)	
Tube well irrigation	75.88% (b)	98.73% (c)	
Canal irrigation	23.20% (b)	01.27% (c)	None (d)
Annual rainfall	465 mm (b)	553 mm (c)	418 mm (d)

Agricultural Yields of the Important Crops in the Three Districts (kg/ha.)***			
Wheat	3530 kg/ha (e)	4256 kg/ha (c) (20.6)	1552 kg/ha(f)
Mustard	1206 kg/ha (e)	1436 kg/ha (c) (19)	-
Bajra	1440 kg/ha (e)	1596 kg/ha (c) (10.8)	586.25 kg/ha (f)

Sources: Information on the number of government health facilities was obtained from the District Action Plan of Mewat (Office of the Civil Surgeon, 2010) and the official websites of Mahendergarh district (Official Website of District Mahendergarh) and Jalore (Official Website of District Jalore) respectively. The literacy levels, household levels, and Maternal and Child care data have been compiled from the DLHS Factsheets of Districts Mewat (GOI, 2007-08 a), Mahendergarh (GOI, 2007-08 c) and Jalore (GOI, 2007-08 d)

a Figure is based on the information obtained from the Office of the Civil Surgeon, Mewat.

b The figures have been taken from the Comprehensive District Agricultural Plans for District Mewat.[7]

c The figures have been taken from the Comprehensive District Agricultural Plan for District Mahendergarh (Singh et al., undated).

d Information obtained from the official website of Jalore district (Official Website of District Jalore).

e These are weighted averages of the yields for each block given in the Comprehensive District Agricultural Plans for District Mewat (Chauhan et al., undated).

f These figures were obtained from the district-wise statistics for different crops provided on the website of the Directorate of Agriculture (2011), Government of Rajasthan.

Note: The economy of all three districts is dependent primarily on subsistence agriculture and allied activities. Availability of water for irrigation is a major problem in all three districts, being worst in Jalore which is a desert area. The situation in Mahendergarh is somewhat better with the district receiving higher rainfall.

The figures in parenthesis are the percentages by which the yield in Mahendergarh is higher than that in Mewat.

– Means the figures are not known.

* The official website of the district mentions that the number of hospitals, dispensaries, and health centres is 132 which is considerably higher than the total figure for Mewat district which has a higher population than Mahendergarh.

**It may be noted that the net cultivable area of Mewat and that of Mahendergarh district is 1, 66,747 ha and 1, 49,374 ha respectively; therefore, even in absolute terms Mewat has a larger irrigated cultivable area.

***The variety of crops grown in Mahendergarh and Jalore is apparently much wider than those grown in Mewat. Only the crops for which yields were available both for Mewat and the other district have been cited here in order to compare agricultural productivity.

The figures in parenthesis are the proportion by which the yield in Mahendergarh is higher than Mewat.

That is not to suggest that better household and health indicators are independent of the prosperity and productivity of agriculture. Mahendergarh district's much higher household standard of living index and maternal and child health service indicators could reasonably be attributed to its considerably higher agricultural productivity (Singh et al., undated) compared to both Mewat and Jalore.

Mahendergarh's higher agricultural productivity cannot be explained only on the basis of the modest advantage it has in terms of annual rainfall received. The irrigated agricultural area is higher in Mewat district both in terms of the proportion of total agricultural area, and also in absolute terms, with canal irrigation being as much as 23.2 per cent of the total irrigation compared to a mere 1.27 per cent for Mahendergarh. Only 35 per cent of Mahendragarh district's ground-water quality is within safe limits for agriculture; in about

25 per cent of the area it is moderately safe, while in the remaining 40 per cent area it is unsafe for consumption in any form (Singh et al., undated). This means that Mahendergarh district does not have any substantial advantage over Mewat district in terms of available water resources to account for the difference in the development indicators of the two districts. Higher agricultural productivity can be the result of various factors such as better agricultural extension services facilitating the adoption of agricultural techniques more suited for the local agro-climatic conditions, better credit facilities for purchase of inputs, and efforts made at improving and restoring soil health. All this can be achieved only if greater attention is paid to the development of an area and its resources.

Marginally better water resources and the resultant increase in agricultural productivity could have played only a partial role in the overall development indicators of Mahendergarh because a comparison between Mewat with Jalore shows that improvement in development indicators can be realized even with poorer water resources and lower agricultural productivity in an area predominantly dependent on agriculture for its sustenance. It can thus be concluded that even though a dearth of water resources and low agricultural productivity have been important reasons for Mewat's lack of development, they do not entirely explain Mewat's backwardness.

Does this then mean that Mewat's backwardness is attributable to lack of physical infrastructure or is it attributable to the backwardness of its people who, because of their reluctance to adopt modern education and a smaller family size under the influence of obscurantist mullahs, have erected barriers to their progress? I have already rejected the latter as a 'victim blaming' approach. Deficiency of infrastructure cannot be accepted as a reason without answering the question of why the infrastructure is so poor in Mewat even compared to other less developed regions?

Is Muslim Majority Status the Stigma of Mewat?

In the entire narrative I have encountered repeated references to 'religious fundamentalism/conservatism' of the Meos as a cause of their backwardness. It needs to be categorically stated that the religion in question here is 'Islam'. I have already rejected this, inasmuch as such expressions amount to a 'victim blaming'; however, we need to be alive to the fact that such expressions also reflect a mindset towards Muslims. Being alive to this in the context of this chapter implies exploring this mindset as the reason for Mewat's backwardness. Indeed, it may be recalled that 'religious beliefs/conservatism' was prominently held out as a reason for the region's backwardness in the narratives of the official establishment while none of the village folk (neither Muslims nor Hindus) mentioned it even once as a cause of their problems.

The prime minister's High Level Committee on the Social, Economic and Educational Status of the Muslim Community of India, popularly known as the Sachar Committee[3] took the lid off the otherwise poorly kept secret of India's social, economic and political reality, that Muslims have been discriminated against in various spheres of life (Government of India, 2006). The Sachar Committee's Report is a watershed inasmuch as it is the first official acknowledgement of the systematic and systemic disadvantage that Muslims in India face as illustrated by their social, economic, and political status vis-à-vis the other socio-religious communities (Government of India, 2006).

Unlike caste discrimination, which has a religious sanction and is acknowledged as such in practice, the practice of discrimination against Muslims is not easily acknowledged, nor may be easily identifiable on the basis of day-to-day examples compared to the practice of untouchability even though we are generally aware of the compartmentalized existence of Muslims vis-à-vis other religious groups in India.

Levelling the allegation of religious discrimination is a sensitive issue and ought not to be made lightly without an empirical basis. I propose here that Mewat's status as a Muslim majority region has been central to its social, economic, administrative, and political neglect, and to substantiate this I shall attempt to argue the case on the basis of hard empirical evidence, much of which has been collated from the Sachar Committee Report.

Muslims constituted 5.8 per cent of the total population in Haryana accoding to the 2001 Census. The proportion of the Muslim population in different districts of Haryana is provided in Table 12. It is evident that the majority of the Muslim population in the state is concentrated in the two districts of Gurgaon and Faridabad. According to the 2001 Census figures, the Muslim population is in these two districts.

Table 12: Proportion of Muslims in the Population of Districts of Haryana

	Districts of Haryana State	*Proportion of Total District Population*
1.	Gurgaon	37.2
2.	Faridabad	11.3
3.	Yamunanagar	10.0
4.	Panipat	6.20
5.	Sonipat	2.30
6.	Karnal	1.80
7.	Jind	1.70
8.	Panchkula	3.90
9.	Hisar	1.10
10.	Ambala	1.70
11.	Bhiwani	0.90
12.	Kurukshetra	1.45
13.	Jhajjar	0.90
14.	Sirsa	0.60
15.	Kaithal	0.70
16.	Fatehabad	0.80
17.	Rohtak	0.60
18.	Mahendragarh	0.40
19.	Rewari	0.40

Source: All India Council for Muslim Economic Upliftment, 2011.

Constituted nearly 71 per cent of the total Muslim population in the state, Mewat district was created by joining the Muslim-dominated areas of Gurgaon and Faridabad districts. Later the Hatin block of Mewat district, with an overwhelming Muslim population, was given over to Palwal district which became the 21st district of the state in 2008 (Official website of Palwal district) The fact that the Muslim population is heavily concentrated in just two districts has important political consequences. According to the electoral calculations of the mainstream political parties, this concentration means that Muslims cease to be the quintessential vote bank beyond the few assembly seats accounted for by these districts, compared to a more homogeneous spread of the Muslim population over a larger number of districts so as to form an electoral constituency capable of tilting the balance in an election. However, if the overall condition of Muslims in India is anything to go by then such considerations have not made much of a difference to the overall welfare of the community. It only means gains for the more influential sections of the community waiting to be co-opted by the political élite. This is not however to deny the fact that the people of Mewat have gained greater political weight through the creation of a separate Mewat district.

Facts Regarding the Socio-Economic Discrimination Against Muslims

The overwhelming concentration of Muslims in Mewat and Palwal districts means that at a macro-level, discrimination against Muslims in Haryana is reflected in the backwardness of Mewat district and Hatin block of Palwal district and vice-versa. As the Muslim population in other districts is under 10 per cent, to document discrimination against Muslims one has to study the socio-economic indicators at the level of villages or cluster of villages. The data presented here suggests discrimination against Muslims exists not only in relation to Mewat but may also exist at the village/locality level in other districts.

Table 13 gives the variation in the incidence of poverty over the years on the basis of the socio-religious categories (SRCs) for a period stretching from 1987-8 up to 2004-5. It is clearly evident that at the national level the incidence of poverty among the Muslims has been higher than that among all Hindus put together both for the rural as well as for urban areas. At the national level as a group, the incidence of poverty among Muslims is less only compared to that among the SCs and STs taken as a group, both in the rural as well as the urban areas.

Haryana being among the more prosperous states in India, the overall incidence of poverty in Haryana, as also that for the separate SRCs, has been much less when compared to the figures for India as a whole both for the rural and urban areas. However, in relation to Muslims, the incidence of poverty among them in Haryana is almost twice that for all Hindus put together both for the rural and urban areas. The slender advantage that Muslims

Table 13: Variation in Incidence of Poverty by Socio-Religious Categories Over Time, 1987-88 to 2004-05

India/Hary.	*Total*			*All Hindus*			*Hindu SCs/STs*			*Other Hindus*			*Muslims*			*Other Minorities*		
	2004-05	*1993-94*	*1987-88*	*2004-05*	*1993-94*	*1987-88*	*2004-05*	*1993-94*	*1987-88*	*2004-05*	*1993-94*	*1987-88*	*2004-05*	*1993-94*	*1987-88*	*2004-05*	*1993-94*	*1987-88*
India (Rural)	28	37	39	28	36	40	41	50	54	21	29	33	33	45	43	18	27	25
Hary. (Rural)	13	28	15	12	26	15	26	45	30	7	18	19	26	53	31	9	33	7
India (Urban)	29	33	38	27	31	36	46	51	55	22	26	32	44	47	53	16	23	27
Hary. (Urban)	21	16	18	21	16	19	40	25	38	16	14	14	46	40	0*	1	23	10

Source: Compiled from 8.5 and 8.6, Appendix, Sachar Committee Report. *This figure seems to be a misprint, but that is how it is given in the original source.

Table 14: Proportion of Villages Having Basic Facilities by Size of Population and by Proportion of Muslim Population

Facility	*India/ Hry.*	*Small (less than 1000 population)*				*Medium (1000 – 2000 population)*				*Large (More than 2000 population)*			
		Within Muslim Population Share of											
		All	*< 9%*	*10-39%*	*40% +*	*All*	*< 9%*	*10-39%*	*40% +*	*All*	*< 9%*	*10-39%*	*40% +*
Education	India	80.4	81.6	71.7	69.4	95.4	96.4	92.4	90.3	98.3	96.7	97.8	96.8
	Hry.	87.1	88.8	79.2	78.6	98.1	98.3	97.6	96.7	99.5	99.5	100	99.3
Health facility	India	20.2	20.2	21.0	19.1	43.5	44.9	39.7	36.0	70.7	73.5	67.2	60.2
	Hry.	23.4	25.4	21.8	8.9	43.1	45.3	47.0	19.8	82.9	83.8	86.7	66.4
Post & Telegraph	India	30.1	30.7	29.4	20.4	54.7	57.5	49.1	36.2	79.8	83.7	76.7	62.2
	Hry.	57.3	60.9	62.4	26.6	70.0	73.0	79.5	35.2	89.4	91.1	85.0	62.9
Busstop	India	28.5	29.1	24.9	23.8	45.0	48.4	33.9	29.2	61.6	67.1	53.1	42.9
	Hry.	59.9	62.0	56.4	44.8	74.5	77.1	59.0	55.5	89.7	90.7	83.3	74.8
Proper approach road	India	45.2	45.1	48.6	42.8	65.5	66.9	63.3	55.4	82.1	84.5	80.7	70.2
	Hry.	97.3	97.5	95.0	97.4	99.3	99.5	97.6	98.9	99.7	99.8	98.3	99.3

Source: Compiled from figures in 7.1 to 7.5, App., Sachar Committee Report.To begin on a more positive note, it needs to be mentioned that more villages in Haryana for every population size and every size of Muslim population in the village, had basic facilities available within the village in compared to the all India figures in the respective categories. Given the fact that Haryana is among the more prosperous of the states with all parts of the state being accessible with relative ease, this finding is not a surprise.

seem to have over the SCs and STs at the national level seems to have been lost by them in Haryana in relation to poverty status. The possible consolation can be that overall decline in the incidence of poverty between 1987-8 and 2004-5 in the rural areas in Haryana has been higher among Muslims at 16 per cent than among the SCs and STs at 13.3 per cent.

The trends cited above are reaffirmed by Table 14 which provides data on the availability of five basic facilities within the village, namely Educational institutions, Health facility, Post and Telegraph facility, Busstop, and an All weather approach road, varying by the size of the village population and the proportion of the Muslim population. All these facilities have a direct bearing on the welfare of the Muslim community either from the perspective of the development of the human capital of the community or from that of facilitating their livelihoods and thereby improving their social and economic position.

Table 15: Gradation in the Availability of Basic Facilities in the Village with the Size of its Muslim Population

Facility	*India/ Haryana*	*Percentage increase in availability from more than 40% Muslim population villages to less than 9% Muslim population villages in the three population categories.*		
		Less than 1000 population	*1000 to 2000 population*	*Over 2000 population*
Education	India	17.6	6.80	-0.1
	Haryana	13.0	1.70	.20
Health facility	India	5.80	24.7	22.1
	Haryana	185.4	128.8	26.2
Post and Telegraph	India	50.5	58.8	34.6
	Haryana	129	107	44.8
Busstop	India	22.3	65.8	56.4
	Haryana	38.4	39.0	21.3
Proper approach road	India	5.40	20.8	20.4
	Haryana	0.10	0.60	0.50

Source: Calculations made by the author based on figures in Tables 13 and 14.

Deriving from Tables 13 and 14, Table 15 mentions the percentage increase in the availability of basic facilities within the village while moving from villages with a 40 per cent + Muslim population to villages with a less than 9 per cent Muslim population in all the three population size categories of villages. Judging by the percentage increase in the availability of education facilities within the village between villages with a 40 per cent + to villages with a 9 per cent Muslim population (Table 15), the bias against Muslims in Haryana is not stronger than that prevalent at the all-India level. However, the differential in availability of health facilities within the village is staggering and much higher than the all India increase between villages with 40 per cent + and 9 per cent Muslim population for all the three village sizes. A similar situation exists in relation to post and telegraph services.

Trends in Educational Achievements of Muslims in Haryana vis-à-vis Other SRCs

The relief that one may experience from the lower negative bias in relation to the all-India figures regarding the availability of educational facilities in Haryana villages with a sizable Muslim population is belied by the figures regarding educational accomplishments of Muslims in Haryana in relation to those at the all-India level. The figures in Tables 16, 17, and 18 clearly show that in relation to overall literacy levels, in proportion of children enrolled (aged 6-14 years.) and in the mean years of schooling of children aged 7 to 16 years, the Muslims have emerged as the least advantaged SRC behind even the SCs and STs. The gap in the mean years of schooling is especially noteworthy in relation to Muslim girls. The mean years of schooling of Muslim girls is likely to be 2.5 times less than that for the SC/ST girls and around 3.5 times less than that for all other SRCs.

Table 16: Literacy Levels by Socio-Religious Categories, India and Haryana, 2001

	All	*Hindus*	*SCs/STs*	*Muslims*	*All Others*
India (13.4)	64.8	65.1	52.2	59.1	70.8
Haryana (5.8)	67.9	69.4	55.4	40.0	72.9

Source: Compiled from Table 4.1, Appendix, Sachar Committee Report. The figures given in the table are estimates from Census of India 2001, Tables C9, C8-SCs, C8-STs. Note: The figures within parenthesis are % share of Muslims in the population.

Table 17: Variance by Socio-Religious Categories in Proportion of Enrolled Children Aged 6-14 Years, India and Haryana

	Total	*SCs/STs*	*H-OBCs*	*H-General*	*Muslims*	*All Others*
All India	85.3	79.7	86.0	94.9	81.8	89.9
Haryana	88.8	79.4	92.1	95.5	59.7	90.6

Source: Compiled from figures in Table 4.3, App., Sachar Committee Report. The estimates in the table are from NSSO 61st round, schedule 10, 2004-5.

Table 18: Mean Years of Schooling of Children Aged 7-16 Years by Socio-Economic Category, 2001

	Group	*Cumulative/Gender-wise*		
		All	*Male*	*Female*
All India	Total	3.95	4.18	3.69
	SCs/STs	3.35	3.67	2.98
	Muslims	3.26	3.40	3.11
	All Others	4.39	4.61	4.15
Haryana	Total	4.33	4.46	4.18
	SCs/STs	3.61	3.79	3.39
	Muslims	2.04	2.63	1.33
	All Others	4.76	4.83	4.67

Source: Compiled from figures in Table 4.2, App., Sachar Committee Report. Estimated from Census of India, 2001, Tables C 9, C 8-SC, C 8-ST.
Note: The age group 7-16 years corresponds to matriculation level of education.

Could it be Accidental?

Some might still contend that these disparities could be purely accidental rather than deliberate. However, the comprehensiveness of these disparities is far too conspicuous to be written off as accidental, and the following example underlines that they are deliberate.

I have already presented a comparison between two most backward districts of Haryana, Mewat and Mahendergarh. Although scarcity of water is a major problem in both the districts, agricultural productivity in Mahendergarh is considerably better than in Mewat. What lies behind this? Table 19 presents a comparison of the outlay for agriculture and allied sectors for both the districts.

Table 19: Comparison of Proposed Outlay for Agricultural Development of Mahendergarh and Mewat Districts for the Eleventh Plan Period (Rs. in Lakhs)

Characteristics	*Mahendergarh*	*Mewat*
Population (2001 census)	813,000	993,000
Rural population	86.51%	92.93%
Percentage of births of order 3 and above	23.1%	57.6%
Total cultivable area	1, 55, 599 hectares	1, 46, 000 hectares
Sector	*Proposed Outlay*	
Agriculture	4999.73	6873.7
Allied sectors	4532.59	1208.85
Total	9532.32	8080.55

Source: Compiled from figures given in Chauhan et al., undated, Singh et al., undated, and DLHS 3 fact-sheets for population figures.

Note: The plan outlay under the Agriculture Sector includes outlay for agriculture, soil conservation, and agriculture engineering, while the outlay for the Allied Sector includes the sub-heads of subsidiary occupations, others, horticulture, animal husbandry, and fisheries.

It is evident from the table that Mewat's population is about 22 per cent larger than Mahendergarh's and the proportion of the rural population is 6.42 per cent higher for Mewat. More importantly, this means that the population dependent on agriculture is larger for Mewat both in absolute and proportionate terms. Moreover, the rate of growth of population is much higher for Mewat than it is for Mahendergarh, which means that the future difference in population is going to be even higher. Add to this the development lag that Mewat suffers compared to Mahendergarh; all these factors put together imply that the requirement of resources for Mewat is much higher than that for Mahendergarh, and yet the allocation for Mewat in the Eleventh Five Year Plan is about 18 per cent less than that for Mahendergarh. That is not saying that the allocation for Mahendergarh should be less, but only to point out the injustice done to Mewat. It is relevant to note that discrimination against Muslims is never announced and yet we can see how it is increasingly pronounced in the Mewat case.

Understanding the Mismatch Between What the People Want and What the Administration Delivers

Just as in the international policy paradigm, it is the developed countries of the north who seem to know what is best for developing countries of the south, within developing countries it is the sophisticated urban and Westernized policy élite who appear to know what is best for the people, rather than taking the cue from the people about what they want. The people invariably are considered to be too simple or ignorant, or downright backward to know what is in their best interest. Again, there is nothing cynical about this at the level of individual public servants; it is reflective more of the governance paradigm prevalent in India.

It should then come as less of a surprise that while the people in Mewat want the problem of water to be redressed first, the Mewat Development Agency's slogan is 'education first'. Within education too, the exclusive priority is on imparting élitist education to barely four per cent of all the students enrolled in Mewat studying in the Mewat Model Schools, while those in the other government schools can make do with the fortuitous incentive of 'midday meals'.

Neither in a country where 52 per cent of the workforce is dependent on agriculture, nor in Mewat where over 90 per cent of the people are directly dependent on agriculture, is education imparted in a way that leads to development in agriculture. The one-sided emphasis on education is directly borne out of the belief that people in Mewat are backward and need to be *'educated'*.

The much promised Mewat Canal Project was cleared by the Planning Commission in 1998. It was to have supplied irrigation water for 2,50,000 acres of land in about 300 villages of the Mewat region (including Hatin block of the newly formed Palwal district) (India Environment Portal, 1998). Following the Planning Commission's approval it was not till 2007 that the Haryana government approved the construction of the 78.74 kms long Mewat Canal at an estimated cost of Rs. 326.40 crores (Bains, 2007). However, to this day not even a brick has been laid for the project. The Haryana Chief Minister Bhupinder Singh Hooda once again promised the Canal to the people of Mewat at a rally held at Nuh on the February 19, 2011; what had changed was that by now the cost of the project has escalated to Rs. 640 crores (*The Hindu*, 2007).

A number of developmental psychologists have proposed different theories regarding the hierarchical nature of human needs. Without going into the specificities of these theories here, at least this much can be reasonably presumed that before a person is able to aspire for a higher quality of life, s/ he ought to have some surety of being able to access his basic physiological needs of food, clothing, and shelter. Mewat has the highest proportion of below the poverty line people in the whole of Haryana and the DLHS 3 survey tells us that it also has the highest proportion of people with a low standard of living. Under conditions in which life is a daily struggle for food and water, illness and the need to access treatment may appear to be a relatively distant possibility. Indeed, even the meaning of illness may change; one wonders how many women in Mewat would consider themselves to be ill because they are severely anaemic. The poor try to cope with ill health till seeking medical care becomes an absolute necessity. Under these circumstances, 'education' may appear to be an even greater luxury, especially as the educated unemployed abound in the area. Is it surprising then that none of the respondents in the household survey at Uleta mentioned good health care and education as being among their priorities. Also, there was considerable wisdom in the statement of one of the respondents that 'once the economic well-being of the people is ensured, they will automatically demand health care and good education'.

This does not however mean that the creation of health infrastructure can wait for now; all that it implies is that the provision of health care must form a part of a composite socio-economic package that is perceptibly seen to be raising the living standards of the people. It is evident that the development process adopted in Mewat has systematically violated every facet of a composite and participatory development process aimed at bringing overall improvement in every aspect of life for a majority of the people.

Concluding Remarks

Any public servant confronted with the kind of data presented above would vehemently deny that s/he is motivated by any bias or discriminates in his or her practice against any person on the basis of caste, creed, or religion. While it may be granted that not every public servant is casteist or communal, it is impossible to ignore that caste and communal privileges run deep in our society. The formally secular structure of our Constitution, legislature, judiciary, and administration only helps to create a smokescreen to cover the communal sentiments that are so rife within the society and the structure of the Indian state.

It is not rare to see that in times of communal crisis the various institutions of the state openly and belligerently acquire communal colours. Every major communal pogrom that India has witnessed in the past few decades has been facilitated with the connivance and even participation of the agencies of the state, be it the anti-Sikh riots following the assassination of the then Prime Minister Indira Gandhi in 1984, the communal riots in various parts of India following the demolition of the Babri Masjid in Ayodhya, the anti-Muslim pogrom in Gujarat in 2002, or even the very recent communal riots in Muzaffarnagar district in western Uttar Pradesh. The chief protagonists of these communal disturbances have ended up occupying positions of power at the Centre and the states, and thereby control and direct state policy.

The dichotomies between words and deeds are numerous and therefore we have an officially and constitutionally mandated reservation policy for oppressed castes and yet every organ of the state assiduously works to ensure its failure in implementation. That Muslims are weighed down with obscurantist religious views is the common refrain, and yet it is only the communal section of the community's leadership that is so enthusiastically cultivated and co-opted by the establishment as a tool to manipulate the Muslim masses. The malady is far too systemic and systematic to be amenable to the sincere efforts of a few public-spirited individuals. The problem fundamentally lies with the present social, economic, and political structure of the Indian state and the way it privileges the fault-lines of caste, class, and religion to maintain its hegemony over the oppressed masses. In the given milieu, even the 'welfare functions' of the state: policies and programmes relating to health, education, women's empowerment, and food security, and the like, become coloured by this dominant character of the state that harbours utter disdain for the people.

Over the years this scheme of things has become so routine and normalized, and people's sensibilities so benumbed, that the latter do not even recognize them as being abnormal. When so much structural violence is ingrained in the system, where is the need for an individual public servant to consciously try and harm a person on the basis of caste, creed, or religion? The truth is that most public servants take this systemic violence as given and normal and therefore fail to question policy. Rather than encourage a rational questioning, the system demands unquestioning compliance. Under the circumstances, finding fault with the people who are the actual victims of underdevelopment becomes a convenient alibi. While the poor development indicators for Mewat may not be the doing of individual public servants working in the district, this does not absolve them of the responsibility to study and understand the systemic causes of the backwardness of the people of Mewat, including discrimination on religious grounds, rather than indulge in victim blaming.

REFERENCES

All India Council for Muslim Economic Upliftment (2011): All India District-wise Muslim Population, Census of India, 2001. Available from: http://www.aicmeu.org/Muslim%20Population%20 Distribution%20in%20India.htm, accessed April 20, 2011.

Bains, S. (2007): 'Haryana Approves Mewat Canal for Rs. 326 Crores', *Punjab Newsline*, March 15. Available from: http://www.punjabnews line.com/share/print/3126, accessed February 10, 2011.

Census of India (2013 a): 'Mewat District: Census 2011 Data'. Available from http://www.census2011.co.in/census/district/226-mewat.html , accessed on November 5, 2013.

Census of India (2013 b): 'Haryana Population Census Data 2011'. Available from http://www.census2011.co.in/census/state/haryana.html accessed on November 5, 2013.

Chauhan, D.R., U.B. Singh, L.S. Yadav (undated): 'Comprehensive District Agriculture Plan for Rashtriya Krishi Vikas Yojana of Eelventh Five Year Plan, Draft Plan, District Mewat, Haryana', Planning Commission, Government of India.

Directorate of Agriculture (2011): 'Rajasthan Krishi', Government of Rajasthan. Available from: http://www.rajasthankrishi.gov.in/ Departments/Agriculture/main.asp?t=statics_top.htm&p =Report

Entry.asp&var=1, accessed April 20, 2011.

Government of India (2009): 'Demographic, Socio-economic and Health Profile of Haryana State as Compared to India', *Haryana State Report*, (New Delhi: National Rural Health Mission, Ministry of Health and Family Welfare).

Government of India (GOI) (2007-8 a): 'District Level Household and Facility Survey under Reproductive and Child Health Project (DLHS-3), fact-sheet Mewat, Ministry of Health and Family Welfare.

Government of India (GOI) (2007-8 b): 'District Level Household and Facility Survey under Reproductive and Child Health Project (DLHS-3), Fact-sheet Haryana, Ministry of Health and Family Welfare.

Government of India (GOI) (2013): 'Provisional Population Totals: India: Census 2011', Ministry of Home Affairs. Available from http://censusindia.gov.in/2011-prov-results/indiaatglance.html accessed on November 5, 2013.

Government of India (2006): Prime Minister's High Level Committee on 'Social, Economic and Educational Status of the Muslim Community of India', Chairman Justice Rajender Sachar (Retd.), November, 2006.

Government of India (2007-8c): 'District Level Household and Facility Survey under Reproductive and Child Health Project (DLHS-3), Fact-sheet Mahendergarh, Ministry of Health and Family Welfare.

Government of India (2007-8d): 'District Level Household and Facility Survey under Reproductive and Child Health Project (DLHS-3), Fact-sheet Jalore, Ministry of Health and Family Welfare.

Institute of Rural Research and Development and Aide et Action (IRRAD) (undated): 'An Assessment of Development Indicators in Rural Mewat'. Available from http://www.smsfoundation.org/links/IRRADAEAACTRESEARCH.pdf accessed on December 2, 2010.

Institute for Human Development (2008): 'A Baseline Survey of Minority Concentration Districts of India, Mewat', Sponsored by the Ministry of Minority Affairs, Government of India & Indian Council for Social Science Research.

Institute of Rural Research and Development (IRRAD) (2010): 'Need Analysis For Gender Equity Training', Capacity Building Centre: Training Need Assessment-Series 1, February. Available from http://www.smsfoundation.org/pdf/Gender-Analysis-Report.pdf accessed on January 5, 2011.

India Environment Portal (1998): 'Planning Commission Clears Mewat Canal Project', January 1. Available from: http://www.india environment portal.org.in/node/127073, accessed February 10, 2011.

Joshi, P. (2003): 'The Cloning of Kamla', *Outlook*, August. Available from http://www.outlookindia.com/article.aspx?221038 and accessed on

December 6, 2010.

Khan, S.A. (2007): Ground Water Information Booklet, Mewat District, Haryana, Central Ground Water Board, Ministry of Water Resources, Government of India.

Mewat Development Agency (2011 a): 'Profile of Mewat'. Available at http://mda.nic.in/Mewat-Profile.htm and accessed on January 23, 2011.

Mewat Development Agency (2011 b): 'Mewat at a Glance'. Available at http://mda.nic.in/Mewat-Glance.htm, and accessed on January 23, 2011.

Mewat Development Agency (2011 c): 'Mewat Model Schools Society, Nuh'. Available from http://mda.nic.in/MMSS.htm and accessed on December, 2010.

Office of the Civil Surgeon (2010): 'District Action Plan, 2010 – 2011', District Mewat.

Official Website of District Mahendergarh, The National Portal of India. Available from http://mahendragarh.gov.in/district_administration.asp#10, and accessed on April 19, 2011.

Official Website of District Jalore. Available from: http://jalore.nic.in/, caccesed on April 19, 2011.

Official Website of district Palwal. Available from: http://palwal.gov.in/ and accessed on April 20, 2011.

Planning Commission (2005): 'Summary Record of the Presentation by Civil Society Groups from Mewat, Haryana', Voluntary Action Cell, Planning Commission, Meeting held on June 30, 2005 at Yojana Bhavan, Planning Commission.

Planning Commission (2011): 'Press Note on Poverty Estimates', Government of India, New Delhi, January.

Planning Commission (2011): 'Report of the Working Group on National Rural Health Mission (NRHM) for the Twelfth Five Year Plan (2012-17)', p. 20.

Sharma, L., Jay Sehgal, Ellora Mubashirand (undated): 'Sustainable Rural Water Management, A Replicable Case Study', The Sehgal Foundation, Gurgaon. Available from www.mgwater.com/ahwa/common_ahwa/doc/iihmrfinalpaper.doc and accessed on December 2, 2010.

Singh, C.P. (2008): 'Feasibility Study of Mobile Medical Unit Operations in Mewat', HelpAge India, Centre for Development of Corporate Citizenship, SP Jain Institute of Management and Research.

Sikand, Y. (1995): 'Meonis of Mewat', *Economic and Political Weekly,* Vol. 30 (10): 490-2.

Singh, V.P., S.S. Yadav, A.S. Yadav, et al. (undated): Comprehensive

District Agriculture Plan, District Mahendergarh, Haryana, Draft Plan under Rashtriya Krishi Vikas Yojana for Eleventh Five Year Plan, Planning Commission, Government of India.

Tribune (2004): 'Call of Mewat', October 24. Available from http://www.tribuneindia.com/2004/20041031/spectrum/main1.htm and accessed on December 3, 2010.

The Hindu (2007): 'Hooda Promises Better Days for Mewat,' February 20. Available from: http://www.thehindu.com/2011/02/20/stories/2011022064420500.htm, cited February 21, 2011.Upadhyay, S. (2007): 'Wastage in Indian Higher Education', *Economic and Political Weekly*, 42 (2), 161-8.

NOTES

1. The findings regarding the district discussed here were made by me as part of the field study of the district health system of Mewat in 2010 when pursuing a Masters in Public Health course from the Centre for Social Medicine and Community Health at Jawaharlal Nehru University, New Delhi. It is also acknowledged that the situation may well have improved in the district since the time of the visit, but subsequent improvements do not prejudice the findings of this report which beget our attention and concern in as much as these reflect the realities of Indian society.
2. The Government of India launched the National Rural Health Mission in 2005 to reinvigorate the rural health services in India. A major policy thrust of the government under the scheme was to increase the proportion of institutional deliveries with a view to providing safe deliveries for the expectant mothers and their newborns to enable the targets for reduction in maternal and infant mortality could be met. In practice, rather than a holistic rejuvenation of health services, NRHM has got skewed in favour of a single-minded focus on maternal and child health, and even so the declared targets of reduction in maternal and infant mortality could not be achieved by the end of the first phase of the mission in 2012.
3. The Committee was constituted under the chairmanship of Justice Rajinder Sachar, former Chief Justice of Delhi High Court.

9

Pay for Performance Programmes in Health Care: An Analysis of Findings from Mewat District in Haryana

Introduction

Provision of monetary incentives for different categories of health workers seems to have become a conventional wisdom for successful implementation of various health programmes. Such is the faith in this strategy that scant effort has been made in India to carefully assess the impact of monetary incentives in the implementation of health programmes, let alone spare attention for the fact that any health programme and health workers have to negotiate a tough social, economic, political and cultural terrain and this may not be so easily circumvented through incentives.

One of the relatively recent health programmes that has been sought to be leveraged through an incentive structure has been the institutional deliveries programme through the JSY (Janani Suraksha Yojana) and the JSSK (Janani Sishu Suraksha Yojana Karyakram) schemes that are components of the central government's flagship health programme—the earlier National Rural Health Mission (NRHM) which has been renamed as the National Health Mission (NHM) after incorporating the National Urban Health Mission in the same programme. This chapter discusses the findings regarding the implementation of institutional delivery scheme in Mewat district to bring out some of the complexities involved in incentive driven programmes and the lessons that derive from it. This study was carried out simultaneously with the study referred to in the earlier chapter.

We may also refer the readers to another of our papers that deals with similar issues regarding the implementation of the JSSK scheme in the state of Uttar Pradesh (Bajpai, 2014).

A Brief Recapitualation of Mewat District

We have already given a detailed profile of Mewat district in the previous chapter and the same need not be gone into over here in detail. We shall only recapitulate very briefly some of the essential facts. Created on April 4, 2005, Mewat is the twentieth district of Haryana state and is located in close proximity to Delhi. The region has a distinct ethno-cultural identity and derives its name from the Meo-Muslims of the region who constitute the predominant population group. Mewat lags far behind the Haryana state average in development indicators.

The health indicators for Mewat are considerably poorer than for the rest of Haryana. The infant mortality rate (IMR) in the district was as high as 85 in Punhana block, which is the largest in the district (Singh, 2008). In comparison, the IMR for Haryana was 58 (95 per cent CI 34-51) in 2008 (RGI, 2009). In 2007-9 the maternal mortality rate for Haryana was 153 (95 per cent CI 90-217) (RGI, 2011). In comparison the maternal mortality in Mewat was estimated to be well above 200 (figure provided by the office of the Civil Surgeon) in 2009-10. Under the circumstances, achieving a sizable reduction in the maternal and infant mortality rates became the highest priority for the district health administration in Mewat.

Further findings and observations presented in this chapter are from the sub-centre at Uleta village in the district. The findings have subsequently been analysed in the context of the available literature in the psychology of motivation to perform as also the general experience of implementation of 'pay for performance' schemes in the health sector.

Need to Lower Maternal and Infant Mortality and the Imperative for Institutional Deliveries

Institutional deliveries have come to be seen as an expedient to achieve expeditious reduction in maternal and infant mortality: two important MDGs (Millennium Development Goals) (RGI and CGHR, 2006). The underlying presumption behind the promotion of institutional deliveries is that 'giving birth in a medical institution under the care and supervision of trained health care providers promotes child survival and reduces the risk of maternal mortality' (Sugathan et al., 2001). Institutional deliveries, it is presumed, besides enabling professional attention, enable the mother to deliver in an appropriate setting where lifesaving equipment and hygienic conditions help in the reduction of the risk of complications that may cause death or illness to the mother and the newborn (Kesterton, 2010). Effective antenatal care is likely to enhance the probability that the mother will deliver in an institution (Sugathan et al., 2001).

India accounts for around 19 per cent of the total global maternal deaths, three-fourths of which occur in just nine Indian states. The government launched the 'Janani Suraksha Yojana' (JSY) (safe motherhood scheme) in April 2005 with the objective of achieving a reduction in maternal and infant mortality by increasing the proportion of deliveries conducted in medical institutions (Dongre, 2010).

Under the JSY a woman is given a monetary reward for delivering in a medical facility, and at the same time community health workers are given performance-linked pay to ensure institutional deliveries for women (Gupta et al., 2012). With the objective of reducing infant and maternal mortality and improving the female sex ratio in the state, the government of Haryana had introduced the Jachcha-Bachcha Scheme on August 15, 2008 that had provisions for providing performance-based cash incentives for encouragment of the ANMs (Auxiliary Nurse Midwife) and the staff nurses to conduct more institutional deliveries in the state. The scheme provided for a cash incentive of Rs 400 for every male child born and Rs 600 for every girl child, after the first three deliveries conducted by the ANM/staff nurse in a month, four weeks after delivery, so as to ensure post-partum and neo-natal care (*OneIndia News*, 2008).

The overriding emphasis on institutional deliveries and incentivization of these led to unprofessional and unethical practices afflicting the implementation of antenatal care and institutional deliveries in the district. This literally cost many infants their lives, resulting in a situation where institutional deliveries were sustaining a high IMR at least in the villages under the Uleta sub-centre.

Turnaround in the Performance of the Uleta Sub-Centre and the Quality of its Services

Till 2006-7 the proportion of institutional deliveries in Uleta village was barely 10 per cent (IRRAD, 2006-7) and till December 2009 there were no deliveries being undertaken at the sub-centre there. The turnaround in the functioning of the sub-centre occurred after it moved to new premises within the village panchayat (council) building and this turnaround is testified to by the impressive rise in the number of institutional deliveries in the villages covered by this sub-centre. Indeed, if the ANMs are to be believed, as on the date of the study very few home deliveries were taking place in the villages under sub-centre Uleta. However, the quality of these 'institutional deliveries' leads us to question whether the avowed objective of reducing the maternal and infant mortality was being achieved. Table 1, given as annexure at the end of the chapter gives the detailed facility survey of the Uleta sub-centre.

Some salient findings of the facility survey for the RCH services are:

- There are two ANMs at the centre and although the nature of work of both are identical, the salary of the permanent ANM is double that of the one working on a contractual basis.
- There is no running water supply available at the sub-centre.
- The electricity supply is variable.
- There is no toilet facility available for the patients or their attendants.
- The blood pressure equipment and haemoglobinometer were non-functional.
- There were no records available to show delivery of post-natal care or newborn care visits.
- The proportion of fully immunized children is only 25 per cent.
- The actual beneficiaries of the JSY scheme make up a very small proportion of the total women who delivered.

These findings are of crucial importance to the quality of care and shall be addressed in greater detail in the subsequent discussion.

Quality of Antenatal Care

Effective antenatal care is the best guarantor of institutional delivery. However, the spurt in the number of institutional deliveries at the Uleta sub-centre is certainly not the result of effective antenatal care as the quality of this leaves much to be desired. Some salient findings regarding antenatal care were:

- Inspection of the antenatal case register showed that barring one or two cases there were no entries under the columns for haemoglobin, blood sugar, urine sugar, urine proteins, and blood pressure. This is not at all surprising as the BP instrument at the centre was dysfunctional and there were no reagents to perform simple blood and urine tests.
- The ANC register showed that most of the cases were being registered at the beginning of the second semester. Most of the ANC cases had a uniform increase of 2 kgs between the weight recorded at the time of registration and the beginning of the third trimester and again an increase of 2 kgs till the time of delivery. Such uniform entries were clearly indicative of gross manipulation.
- The entries in the columns for the first and the second dose of tetanus toxoid injections were also irregular, though it is difficult to comment on whether this was on account of the mother not having taken the dose or because of irregular maintenance of the register.
- At least for the months of September, October, November, and the first half of December 2010 there was no entry suggestive of pre-eclampsia such as swelling of the feet, headache, or visual disturbances for any antenatal case; nor was there any other complication indicated such as bleeding per vagina (bleeding from vagina).

The findings of the antenatal register were triangulated by assessing the theoretical knowledge of the ANMs which was on the whole fair. For example, to the pointed question of how much weight gain should occur during pregnancy, their reply was: around 8 kgs. This however does not explain the entries of weight recorded in the antenatal register for different trimesters, but then diligence is the first casualty of a slackening in the standards of care.

Nevertheless, sound knowledge can hardly compensate for unsound practice. The above observations regarding antenatal care together with lack of crucial facilities such as running water, regular electricity supply, irregular supply of consumables, and poor or entirely non-existent post-natal and neonatal care and a woefully small proportion of fully immunized children, raise serious questions regarding the overall quality of services being provided by the sub-centre. In this context, the remarkable increase in the number of institutional deliveries being conducted at the sub-centre seems to have less merit and appears to have come at the cost of quality care.

Quality of Institutional Deliveries

While the district administration does emphasize its priorities in terms of improving the quality of antenatal care and increasing the proportion of fully immunized children besides improving the number of institutional deliveries, as regards the ANMs at the Uleta sub-centre, the incentive-linked institutional deliveries seem to have brought out the daring in them with less care for safety.

Given its development profile and the fact that the overall maternal and infant mortality for Mewat is considerably higher than that of Haryana as a whole, we can expect more pregnancy-related complications among the women. The poor quality of antenatal care at the Uleta sub-centre added to our suspicion that this was the case. The ANMs are not supposed to attend to any complicated deliveries; however, inspection of the delivery register at the sub-centre did not reveal a single case being referred from the sub-centre to a higher level medical institution on account of any pregnancy-related complication. The ANMs at the sub-centre proudly proclaimed that except for one case in which there was a hand presentation, not a single delivery case has been referred from their centre to the PHC or the General Hospital at Mandi Kheda over the last year. This case too was referred only because the ANMs were preoccupied with a special campaign for measles vaccination.

This was most surprising and my enquiry revealed some

interesting and worrisome facts regarding the way institutional deliveries were being practised at the sub-centre. The ANMs themselves said that:

- A delivery case is entered in the delivery register only when the delivery has been successfully performed.
- In the eventuality of there being some complication with the delivery, the case is referred to the higher level facility without this being entered in the register, and therefore there are no referrals on record.

Ostensibly, Uleta is not the only sub-centre that follows this practice because another ANM posted at the Bhadas sub-centre also reported a similar practice. The reason given by the ANMs for this is that in the event of the woman's attendants insisting on the patient being referred to a higher institution, then 'our efforts would go waste' if the patient's name was entered as soon as she arrived at the centre with labour pains. This would also necessitate their having to explain the circumstances of the referral to their superiors.

The LHV (Lady Health Visitor) at PHC, Nagina, who is supposed to supervise the ANMs, admitted that this is an irregular practice which continues even though the ANMs have been told not to engage in it. To the question of whether any action had ever been taken against the erring ANMs, the answer was: 'That is not possible; when senior officials are themselves not bothered, what can I do at my level?'

A more detailed discussion with a paediatrician at the district hospital, who had spent over 15 years in the state's health service, helped us to understand the real reasons better. The facts of this practice, as they emerged, are:

- As a result of the *jacha-bacha* scheme a trend had developed among the ANMs throughout the state to first attempt delivering a woman themselves, including complicated cases involving a bad obstetric history, a previous caesarian section, severe anaemia, abnormal placenta, pre-eclampsia or foetal distress. Such cases are more frequently associated with complications that can endanger the life of the mother or the baby or both.

- If the delivery is successful they then register the case in the delivery register as a marker of higher performance in terms of higher institutional deliveries and also ensuring monetary gains that come with the Jachcha-Bachcha scheme.
- If there is any complication midway in the delivery, then the woman's relatives can be asked to go to a higher institution without having to show a formal referral. More importantly, they do not have to shoulder any responsibility for botching up the case in any way as in the absence of any record the woman's family has no way of proving that the delivery was attempted at the centre where it should not to have been attempted at all.
- The comment by the ANMs that 'our efforts would go waste' need be understood as follows: if for some reason during the progress of the labour the woman's attendants do not feel confident that the ANMs are equal to the task and apprehending risk to woman's or baby's life they insist on taking the woman elsewhere, then the effort that the ANMs would have put into the delivery would go waste.
- There is limited accountability sought in the system for post-partum care and monitoring of the mother or the baby for possible adverse consequences. Neither do most of the delivery points have the facilities to keep the mother and the baby for 48 hours to monitor post-partum recovery, nor do the relatives wish to keep the mother and baby for that long in the institution after delivery. This creates impediments in the management of post-partum complications in the mother or the baby.

The overarching drive to increase the number of institutional deliveries ensures a level of tolerance for such practices to the detriment of the safety of the mother's and the baby's life. Table below gives the delivery and infant mortality statistics of the sub-centre. No maternal deaths were reported from the villages falling under the purview of the sub-centre for the past year.

Table : Delivery Statistics and Infant Deaths at Uleta Sub-Centre in 2010

Indicator	*Measure*
Total number of ANC cases registered in 2010	349
Total births under Uleta sub-centre	306
• Institutional deliveries	244 (of these 217 took place at the Uleta sub-centre)
• Home deliveries	62
Total infant deaths	26

Source: Information obtained through the medical officer in charge of Nagina PHC which supervises the Uleta sub-centre.

The total infant deaths in 2010 were 26. The total live births reported in the villages falling within the purview of the sub-centre in 2010 were 306. This would translate into an IMR of 85 per thousand live births and the percentage of institutional deliveries being nearly 80 per cent. Such a high IMR is just not acceptable by any standards. Incidentally, this is also equal to the aforementioned worst estimates for IMR in the district reported from Punhana block.

As regards maternal mortality too there is reason for alarm even though no maternal mortality was reported in the villages falling under the purview of the sub-centre. Table shows the total number of ANC cases registered in 2010 to be 349; however, the total number of births, both institutional and home, has been only 306; this means that 43 ANC cases need to be accounted for. This number cannot be accounted for by abortions because the practice at the sub-centres under PHC Nagina (and probably the whole of Mewat or even Haryana) is to register a woman in ANC clinics only in the fourth month. The reason given by the ANMs for this practice is that some of the women prefer to abort on account of sex selective abortion and therefore if they register the woman in the first trimester and she gets an abortion done, then they will need to account for the abortion to their superiors, which is an unnecessary hassle. That 43 women migrated out of the six villages under the sub-centre is implausible and the total of 306 deliveries in the villages under the purview of the sub-centre includes the institutional as well as home deliveries performed outside those villages, i.e. outside the sub-centre's purview.

What makes matters all the more curious is that the ANMs refused to part with the names of the women who had delivered at the sub-centre during the last month; in fact the ANMs were visibly hostile to the questions, especially those relating to deliveries and antenatal care. The data cited in Table 4 could only be obtained through the active intervention of the medical officer in charge of the Nagina PHC.

The sub-centre does not have any lifesaving equipment to ensure safe deliveries for the mother and the baby. A suction machine is unavailable in the event of the need for emergency suction in cases of foetal distress. There is no arrangement for keeping the newborn babies warm; the bedding to keep the baby warm has to be brought by the woman's relatives and if the paediatrician at the district hospital is to be believed, in rural areas of Haryana people receive only those clothes for receiving the baby post-delivery which are to be discarded as the baby is considered to be unclean immediately after birth.

The number of beneficiaries under the NRHM component of the JSY comprise 6.2 per cent of the total deliveries, while the beneficiaries under the state component (*Jacha-Bacha* scheme) is even less at 2.3 per cent. The payment for the beneficiary mothers has also been delayed by several months, e.g. those who had their delivery in January, received the money only in December. The modality of payment by cheque is also inconvenient for some as in a place where the poor generally do not have any dealing with banks, the women are even more unlikely to have bank accounts in their name. The expenditure incurred on getting an account opened, further reduces the marginal benefits of the scheme.

Social Orientation and Understanding about NRHM of the Sub-Centre Health Workers

Much of the development of health infrastructure that has taken place in Mewat over the past two or three years has been possible only due to the launching of the NRHM. One would then expect the health workers to have been imparted some understanding of the aims and objectives and the strategies of the mission. However, not surprisingly, there was a profound lack of such an orientation among the health workers at Uleta. The ANMs were barely aware of what NRHM stood for and what it sought to achieve, or what the core strategies of the mission were. There was no understanding too of inter-sectoral coordination, the importance of panchayati raj institutions and why there was a need for active participation of the people in such bodies.

At least an understanding of these issues would enable the ANMs to activate the institutional mechanisms such as the VHND and VHSC (Village Health and Sanitation Committee) in order to fully utilize them. But here we had a situation where the energy of the ANMs was single-mindedly focused on RCH-related activities of 'institutional deliveries' and 'immunization'. Though the VHSC exists in Uleta village its functioning is quite ad hoc; the orientation is not towards planning for village health but to get some of the more expedient tasks done.

Even though the ASHA is the key figure for activating village health care under NRHM, the ASHA at Uleta did not seem to be aware that she owes her position to the NRHM. Some of the important aspects of NRHM such as the 'Total Sanitation Campaign' and 'Safe Drinking Water' have remained outside the purview of the work of the sub-centre. As a result of all this, as we shall see later, the sub-centre's activities have failed to touch the lives of the common villager and the villagers remain rather indifferent to its functioning.

Discussion

The moot question here is whether the 'pay for performance incentives' are a desirable method for increasing the coverage of health services in pursuit of public health goals. More specifically, should implementation of health schemes be powered by monetary incentives? Answering these questions requires a nuanced understanding of the issues involved.

Health is a social good and is essential for human well-being. For the poor it is especially important in order to face the multifarious disadvantages of poverty. It can then be reasonably expected that on the demand side there should be a willingness on part of the people, especially the poor, to embrace health services and on the supply side a willingness on part of the health personnel to provide these services effectively and efficiently considering their importance for society's development. However, the present state of the delivery of health services and their utilization by the people is far from desirable. This raises the question of the barriers to the provisioning and the utilization of health services. Inter-alia, under what conditions will the people be motivated to optimally use the health services and the health care providers in turn to be motivated to make these services available to the people. In sum, what are the motivational factors for both to act in conjunction to improve the health of society?

We shall attempt to understand these questions by a two-pronged approach first by examining the systemic factors that either act as an impediment to or as a catalyst for the utilization and provisioning of health services, and second, by examining the theories of motivation.

The Systemic Factors

The supply and the uptake of health services is mediated through the agency of the given social, economic, and political structure of the society and its associated cultural moorings which determine the behaviour of the health care providers and the health-seeking behaviour of the people. There can be different factors: Social (discrimination on the basis of caste, class, race, religion, or gender); economic (lack of purchasing power), physical (lack of health facilities, deficiency of health manpower, difficult topography); political (lack of commitment of governments to health care and other social services); and cultural (lack of education leading to lack of knowledge and superstitions or cultural beliefs regarding particular kinds of services or class and cultural background of the health care providers themselves), that act as barriers in the delivery and utilization of health services. Each one of these factors is related to different dimensions of the overall socio-economic development of the people.

These barriers are not mutually exclusive but are in a dynamic relationship with one another, meaning thereby that action in relation to one also invariably impacts on other factors. This implies that improving the health of the people demands action in relation to each of these factors which affect different aspects of the socio-economic development of people. The Alma Ata Declaration of 1978 was categorical in stating that 'Economic and social development, based on a New International Economic Order, is of basic importance to the fullest attainment of health for all' (WHO, 1978). The declaration went on to state that Primary Health Care 'involves, in addition to the health sector, all related sectors and aspects of national and community development, in particular agriculture, animal husbandry, food, industry, education, housing, public works, communications and other sectors; and demands the coordinated efforts of all those sectors' (WHO, 1978).

Therefore, to positively impact the complex dynamics of the impediments to the delivery and utilization of health services cited above it is necessary that the organization, delivery, and utilization of health services are conceptualized as forming part of the overall development strategy. More importantly, the development strategy should take into account the aspirations of the people in general and more specifically the epidemiological needs in relation to the development of health services. Such an approach would lead to the more holistic objective of promoting 'maximum community and individual self-reliance and participation in the planning, organization, operation and control of primary health care, making fullest use of local, national and other available resources' (WHO, 1978).

Intuitively speaking, a strategy for development and implementation of health services that successfully elicits people's participation in the 'planning, organization, operation and control' of health services meant for their own use would also succeed in eliciting their enthusiasm to ensure the achievement of the public health goals that are sought to be achieved through these services. It would seem unlikely that under such circumstances the health-care providers would be able to shirk their responsibility in delivering these services, not necessarily because of the policing oversight of the people but because such a development paradigm would of necessity entail that all the genuine needs of the health-care providers would also be fulfilled with the active cooperation of the people.

This should then obviate the need to institute financial 'inducements' for people to use the services and for the providers to provide them. In reverse, a development paradigm that alienates the people from exercising control over or demanding answerability from the health services that are meant for them would engender amongst them a measure of detachment from these services, except in unavoidable circumstances. When this happens there can be a loosening of commitment on part of the health care providers to serve the people with dedication. This can lead to a mismatch between the priorities and the needs of the providers and the consumers of health services.

Regrettably, the development paradigm that has been pursued in India since independence, and more specifically since 1990 when neoliberal economic reforms were initiated, has undermined the kind of integrated development of health services described above. It is such development trajectories that the governments and policy-makers seek to impose on the people with their own priorities by projecting them as serving the best interest of the latter without regard to what people desire for themselves. There is even a tendency to suggest that the people themselves are incapable of judging where their best interest lies and that therefore the 'more knowledgeable' experts should determine this for them.

Not only are programmes and schemes rolled out in accordance with governmental priorities, but even targets are determined for their implementation. The vertical disease-control programmes as against strengthening of the general health systems for integrated management of public health problems, the massive target-oriented family planning programme that wreaked havoc on the development of general health services for years, the imposition of DOTS (directly observed therapy short course), an obsession with increasing the rates of institutional deliveries in order to reduce maternal and infant mortality as the core strategy of NRHM without regard to the provision of these services as part of comprehensive health care services and addressing the need to tackle the larger social determinants of health are just some examples of the government's lopsided health schemes.

Such health programmes/schemes catch the imagination of neither the people nor the health care workers. It is perhaps in recognition of the lack of active uptake of these services by the people and participation of health care personnel that monetary incentives have been built into the system. The question is whether such incentives sufficiently motivate the users and the providers.

People's Motivation: Evidence from Psychology

Simply expressed, motivation implies that a person is energized or activated into doing a particular thing or towards achieving a particular end (Ryan and Deci, 2000a). It is also recognized that 'most people show considerable efforts, energy and commitment in their lives appears in fact, to be more normative than exceptional, suggesting some very positive and persistent features of human nature' (Ryan and Deci, 2000b). The levels of motivation amongst people and also differences in motivation between them are ignited by their social contexts and environments, and therefore people are more motivated and energized in certain social contexts, environments, situations, or cultures than in others (Deci and Ryan, 1985, 1991; Ryan, 1995). It would follow from this that to work and to engage in socially useful activity is a fundamental human need and that the challenge is to provide societal conditions in which people can realize this need.

Classical literature in psychology recognizes two types of motivations: intrinsic and extrinsic (Ryan and Deci, 2000a; Ryan and Deci, 2000b; Covington and Mueller, 2001; Lepper et al., 1997). deCharms recognizes extrinsic motivation to be 'pale and impoverished' (even if a potent) when contrasted with intrinsic motivation (deCharms, R. (1968).

Intrinsic Motivation

Cultures around the world attach significance to the distinction between whether people engage in a particular form of behaviour or activity because they attach positive values to such behaviour or for reasons extrinsic to their persona (Johnson, 1993). (The former is identified as 'intrinsic motivation' and is identified with the natural desire among all human beings to explore, to gain mastery over new things, and to assimilate them as their own; features that impart meaning to people's lives and are important to their cognitive and social development (Csikszzentmihalyi (?) and Rathunde, 1993; Ryan, 1995). Deci and Ryan, 1985 propounded the 'Cognitive Evaluation Theory' (CET) which postulated that 'intrinsic motivation, being inherent, will be catalysed when individuals are in conditions that conduce towards its expression'. In other words, if provided with favourable circumstances, the people's natural desire to perform will prosper.

Taking into cognizance the evidence from experimental psychology regarding effects of rewards, positive or negative feedback, and other external factors on internal motivation, CET recognizes that a sense of 'competence' and 'autonomy' are the psychological needs that strengthen 'internal motivation' (Ryan and Deci, 2000 b) to perform a task. For example, a positive feedback is likely to enhance an individual's perception of his competence and thereby his 'internal motivation' to perform a task (Deci, 1975; Vallerand and Reid, 1984). Drawing on the work of Fischer, 1978; Ryan, 1982; and deCharms, 1968, CET further specifies that a sense of enhanced competence alone is not sufficient to enhance 'internal motivation' unless accompanied also by a sense of 'autonomy' . That is, people need to feel that their behaviour is self-determined, free of any external coercion or inducement to experience 'intrinsic motivation'. This implies that to elicit people's 'internal motivation' for positive behaviour that impacts their social and economic development, we need societal conditions that will enhance individual and collective competence to perform the task and the task itself will be so planned that it takes into account their specific needs and desires and thereby endows them with a sense of self-determination/autonomy in the accomplishment of the task.

Evidence from various sources suggests that 'extrinsic rewards' invariably work towards undermining 'intrinsic motivation' of people (Deci, 1975; Deci, Koestner and Ryan, 1999) although there are some dissenions to this view (Eisenberger and Cameron, 1996).

Further research has shown that 'intrinsic motivation' abounds in social contexts that assure people of a sense of security and relatedness. For example, a study by Anderson, Manoogian, and Grolnick (1986) found that left to perform an interesting task in the presence of an apathetic adult stranger, the children demonstrated a very low level of internal motivation. Similarly, Ryan and Grolnick (1986) observed that disinterested and uncaring teachers evoked limited intrinsic motivation amongst their students. In the context of implementation of health programmes these observations would imply that a strategy of providing active support and encouragement to the people and prioritizing their initiatives is most likely to help governments to arouse the internal motivation of the people to participate wholeheartedly in the successful implementation of health programmes.

In sum, the framework of CET suggests that the societal conditions/environments/circumstances of the people can either motivate or defuse the 'intrinsic motivation' of people in the accomplishment of a task by either satisfying or negating their psychological needs. Among these needs the need to enhance the sense of a feeling of competence and autonomy is central and this can be further supported by satisfaction of the need for relatedness. However, above all, 'intrinsic motivation' can only be forthcoming for activities that are of innate interest to the people; activities that satisfy their urge for novelty, challenge, and aesthetic value.

Extrinsic Motivation and its Self-Regulation

Ryan and Deci have defined 'extrinsic motivation' as the 'performance of an activity in order to attain some separable outcome' (Ryan and Deci, 2000b). This is in sharp contrast to 'intrinsic motivation' which implies 'doing an activity for the inherent satisfaction of the activity itself' (Ryan and Deci, 2000b).

The complexity of real-life situations may seldom present situations where the motivation to perform a task may be purely intrinsic. Indeed, in much of the life beyond childhood a person often feels obliged to engage in activities and assume responsibilities that might be of the least interest to him/her (Ryan and La Guardia, 2000).

The practical question that needs to be answered here is what motivates people to engage in 'non-intrinsically' motivated activities and what is the qualitative impact of this motivation on their behaviour and well-being? Ryan and Deci, 2000b, have sought to answer this through their 'Self-Determination Theory' (SDT).

In situations where extrinsically motivated behaviour is sought to be induced in people their response can vary from a total lack of motivation, to passive adherence, to active indulgence. To quote Ryan and Deci, SDT implies that:

> Different motivations reflect differing degrees to which the value and regulation of the requested behaviour have been internalized and integrated. Internalization refers to people "taking in" a value or regulation, and integration refers to the further transformation of that regulation into their own so that, subsequently, it will emanate from their sense of self (Ryan and Deci, 2000b).

Further, SDT addresses two issues (Ryan and Deci, 2000b):

a) The processes through which such non-intrinsically motivated behaviour can become truly self-determined and
b) The ways in which the social environment influences those processes.

Practical Significance of SDT

SDT has practical significance in situations where the health-seeking behaviour of the people or the behaviour of health care providers is sought to be modulated through external inducements. For example, in a pay for performance health service health workers may perform the service because non-performance would lead to financial loss or because they realize its value for career progression. In both cases, instrumentality is external to the inherent pleasure and satisfaction of engaging in the work itself and yet, while the former case involves submitting to external regulation, the latter implies personal endorsement and choice. The two types of behaviour vary in their relative autonomy.

It is however important to note that the act of performing the service has been alienated from the more desirable virtue of 'performing the service for the joy and for its inherent value'. Also, as SDT implies, there are processes whereby 'non-intrinsically motivated behaviour can become truly self-determined' and that these processes can be enhanced by the application of appropriate social environmental influences.

For example, in an overall scenario of large-scale commercialization of health care, 'pecuniary gain' becomes the overriding conscious motive of health care providers. Even for medical students, rather than a keen interest in medicine and a desire to serve humanity, the prospects of a lucrative career becomes the motive force. Thus, as a consequence of a commercialized social environment, providing treatment primarily with the objective of making money becomes the 'self-determined' behaviour of health-care providers.

By contrast, health services can be so organized that they are provided free of commercial motives and the delivery of health-care is considered to be a social good, fulfilment of which is essential to ensuring human welfare. Under such conditions, provided health services fulfil the felt or epidemiological needs of the consumers while ensuring their physical, social, and economic access, and the material requirements of the health care providers for a reasonable standard of living are fulfilled, provision of health services can command an inherent value and provide inherent pleasure.

'Pay for Performance' (P4P) in Health Programmes

Performance incentives became a singular feature of health care delivery in the developed countries of the West during the 1990s with programmes rewarding both the process indicators and qualitative clinical outcomes (Rosenthal et al., 2004). Interestingly, it was concern for low quality of care notwithstanding the high cost to the system that led insurance companies to institute the 'Pay for Performance' (P4P) schemes in health, to begin with, in the UK and the USA (Ryan and Werner, 2013; Abduljawad and Al-Assaf, 2011). In the low and middle income countries, P4P schemes were introduced in the late 1990s and have mushroomed since (Franco, Bennett and Kanfer, 2002). These facts have an important bearing on this discussion inasmuch as they tell us that P4P health programmes are typically a market-oriented solution to improving the quality and efficiency of health programmes. Market-oriented solutions, on the strength of inherent quality, would view people's motivation to perform, even intrinsically motivating services such as health care in purely monetary terms. This means that such solutions are incapable of leveraging people's 'intrinsic motivation' except by strengthening the processes that assist the internalization of 'extrinsic rewards' as self-motivated. P4P solutions would then in general run counter to the more holistic approach of 'Primary Health Care' as delineated above as the latter is possible only by strengthening publicaly funded health care and by curbing the role of markets in health care.

Drawing upon the logic of performance pay in human resource

management, P4P incentives emphasize rewards for health service providers upon fulfilment of pre-specified health targets (Hall and Liebman, 1998; Lazear, 2000). Rewards are a form of recognition and recognition of efforts inculcates a sense of loyalty among employees, which in turn leads to dedication in work (Abduljawad and Al-Assaf, 2011). Abduljawad and Al-Assaf set out two goals to be achieved through carefully instituted customized rewards for employees: 'sparking an interest or change in behaviour' (Abduljawad and Al-Assaf, 2011):

1. For a motivated performance or to enable them to continue to perform better.
2. To achieve a long lasting impact on their performance.

The question is however: What has been the experience of P4P schemes vis-à-vis the achievement of these goals? While a comprehensive review is beyond the scope of this chapter, we feel reasonably confident in stating that evidence regarding a gainful impact of P4P schemes is somewhat ambiguous. Summarizing the world-wide experience of P4P health programmes, Wilson writes: 'Despite broad international experience with pay-for-performance, evidence of its impact is limited, frequently conflicting, focuses largely on improvements in the provision and structure of care rather than health outcomes, and tends to generate more questions than it does answers' (Wilson, 2013). In another thorough review of international evidence on P4P systems published in 2006, the authors have concluded that there have been few, if any, positive net outcomes for health systems as a result of P4P schemes. To the contrary such arrangements were found to have generated a 'perverse incentive' and their implementation was fraught with high costs on account of their complex designs and administration (Golden, 2006).

A custom-made market-oriented solution could have been expected to work better in the market-driven health care system of the US. However, it is astonishing that there is scant evidence to show that P4P has produced an improvement in the quality of American health care. It is further suggested that rather than motivating the desired behaviour, these policies may be encouraging cheating and other unintended behaviour (Ryan and

Werner, 2013). There is no evidence to show improvement in patient outcomes, and even when health care providers have responded favourably to P4P, the response has been focused narrowly on the outcomes that were incentivized, to the detriment of other outcomes (Ryan and Werner, 2013). Another study from the primary care setting in the US found that the physician P4P programme did not lead to any improvement in the quality of preventive care (Gavagan et al., 2010).

The National Health Service (NHS) of the UK did indeed roll out a quite well-structured 'Quality and Outcomes Framework' in which the bonuses to be earned by the general physicians were linked to a comprehensive range of quality indicators. One study analysed longitudinal data from the study to record that if financial incentives led to a neglect of activities they were not incentivized. It was found that the improvements recorded in the incentivized outcomes came at the expense of 'small detrimental effects' for outcomes that were not incentivized (Doran et al., 2011).

Some of the arguments that are advanced in support for P4P incentives are that in primary/rural health care setting monetary incentives help to achieve specific programmatic objectives within a specified time as the Community Health Workers (CHWs) can be pushed to work longer hours. Monetary incentives may facilitate stricter supervision of health workers, rapid implementation of programmes, standardization of work routines, and maintenance of service quality (Phillips, 1999). Monetary incentives also facilitate longer retention of community health workers (CHWs) (Gray and Ciroma, 1987; Wubneh, 1999). To say the least, these measures reflect an attitude of coercive rather than supportive supervision over health workers and may well be a poor expedient for short-term success but are most definitively inappropriate as a means of inculcating dedication and commitment amongst health workers with the aim of achieving public health goals.

It must however be admitted that had there been no successes with P4P programmes there would have been no necessity for such a lengthy discussion. P4P programmes have led to a marked improvement in health outcomes in several projects in different locations. For example, even small monetary incentives for poor and very poor families in the Bolse Familia programme in Brazil are reported to have led to increased participation of these families in health programmes and led to a decrease in poverty levels, decrease in child mortality, and improvements in maternal health (Lindert, 2005). Similar conditional cash transfer schemes for nearly 11 million families were implemented elsewhere in Latin America in 2006 as part of a project to achieve Millennium Development Goals. Appreciable improvements were noticed in child nutrition, improvements in school attendance, immunization, etc. (World Bank, 2004).

Other examples include reduction in anaemia among Chinese schoolchildren through incentives offered to primary school principles (Miller et al., 2012); monetary rewards caused Indian day care workers to devise innovative ways of reaching out to the affected families besides providing nutritious meals in the facilities and thereby resulting in a reduction in malnutrition (Singh, 2011); improvements were noticed in the uptake of services for prenatal care and institutional deliveries in Rwanda (Rusa et al., 2009; Basinga et al., 2011 and Gertler and Vermeersch, 2012), and similarly in prenatal and child care services in Nicaragua (Regalia and Castro, 2009).

Continuing delivery of quality health services in accessibility entails developing stable health institutions and systems in which the greatest incentive attached to the provisioning of health services is that it fulfils an important societal need and the greatest incentive for their utilization is the need to keep the body disease free. This cannot be done in perpetuity if health care is dispensed in a project mode. Even if we were to discount the fact that most of the aforementioned success stories come from studies supported by neoliberal institutions (the World Bank and the Washington DC-based Centre for Global Development) which would have a propensity to support market-oriented solutions, it needs to be noted that these successes were scored through services delivered by different projects. What one needs to know further more about these projects is their long-term sustainability, especially as these involve long-term financial commitment to continue providing monetary incentives; what is the impact of such projects on the more important concerns regarding the long-term development of health services?

There is a paucity of literature dealing with such questions; however, there are studies to show that there could be reasons for concern. Leading management scholar, W. Edward Deming demonstrated that efforts to invoke individual motivation in situations where systematic effort is required is ill-founded. Deming demonstrated that efforts to build the performance of each individual worker would not lead to an improvement in the overall system and stressed the need to improve the performance of the entire system (Abduljawad and Al-Assaf, 2011).

There are a host of unintended outcomes associated with incentive schemes which cause them to become a double-edged sword. For example, incentivizing successful treatment of a disease could undermine efforts to prevent it. Given the importance of 'impact evaluation', especially with regard to the evaluation of individual programmes, there could be a disproportionate shifting of effort to improve primary outcomes, away from the secondary outcomes, as this is what would ensure continued funding of the project or health programme (Miller and Babiarz, 2013). There could be 'cherry-picking' of patients when incentivizing good patient outcomes leading to neglect of sicker and more remote patients (Shen, 2003; Oxman and Fretheim, 2008). Financial incentives could undermine the trust between patients and providers (Ellingsen and Johannesson, 2008). There is also some evidence to suggest that P4P programmes may even increase inequalities in health (Victoria et al., 2000; Doran et al., 2008; Ashworth et al., 2007).

Above all, 'extrinsic rewards' could undermine the 'intrinsic motivation' to perform tasks (McDonald et al., 2007; Ashraf, Bandiera, and Jack, 2012). Even if there are short-term gains, the impact of financial rewards on intrinsic motivation remains an important long-term concern.

Social psychologists have hypothesized that extrinsic rewards impact upon an individual's perception of themselves, the value of the rewarded task (Gneezy, Meier, and Rey-Biel, 2011), and the social perception of the task (Gneezy and Rustichini, 2000). These could be the reasons behind experimental observations that individuals offered monetary incentives to perform tasks that are intrinsically motivating put in considerably less effort in performing the task when incentives are withdrawn (Deci, Koestner, and Ryan,

1999; Kamenika, 2012). One can only imagine the consequences of this for the general health services on the performance of health workers after the financial rewards are discontinued from a health programme.

That monetary incentives are fraught with the risks outlined above does not however mean that there are no valid ways of rewarding health care providers for effort that makes them stand apart from others. There is considerable literature attesting to the virtues and the desirability of non-financial incentives (Franco, Bennett, and Kanfer, 2002; Benabou and Tirole, 2003; Maung et al., 2006; Tonin and Vlassopoulos, 2012; Amare, 2011; Bhattacharya et al., 2001). This is however accompanied by a caveat that the genuine material needs of health workers must be met and the system ought to find the resources to fulfil these needs.

Applying the Findings to the Mewat Situation

We noticed above that despite a very high proportion of institutional deliveries of 80 per cent, the infant mortality for the Uleta sub-centre for the year 2010 was as high as 85 per 1000 live births. We do not have previous figures for IMR in the villages served by the sub-centre for comparison, but the observed proportion of institutional deliveries at the sub-centre was higher than that for Delhi at 69 per cent and yet the IMR for Delhi was much lower than that for Uleta at 25.44 in 2007. This IMR for Delhi represented an increase from an IMR of 12.89 in 2005 (Directorate of Economics and Statistics, 2010). Even though the proportion of institutional deliveries increased from 65.1 per cent in 2005-6, to 71.2 per cent in 2007-8 (NIHFW, 2010). These findings show that there is no direct correspondence between the proportion of institutional deliveries and IMR nor are the assumptions of an enhanced quality of deliveries conducted in institutions necessarily true.

As to the findings at the Uleta sub-centre, one may say that the deliveries could have been conducted very safely, and that the ANMs cannot be blamed if the post-delivery infant care and nutrition are wanting for reasons of poverty or because the mother is burdened with household and farm work which leave less time for her to care for the baby. Well, that's precisely the point; if the government is serious about reducing the IMR and the MMR, it has to go beyond the narrow techno-centric approach or the temptations of shortcuts when sustainable improvement in health is essentially a function of comprehensive development that secures the nutritional, educational and economic security of the people.

In the policy establishment there seems to be an obsession with 'quick fixes'; if old ones fail, find new ones. Moreover, in practice, quick fixes come across as an alternative to more systemic changes; they draw attention away from even what is relatively easily doable under the circumstances. In the case in point, even though institutional deliveries have risen, the post-delivery home visits to care for the health of the mother and the baby is poor, but the indicator for which answerability might be sought is 'institutional delivery' and not the standards of post-natal care. We therefore have a situation where a high proportion of institutional deliveries have ended up achieving the least desirable results. This is indeed a tragic commentary on the incentive-led growth of institutional deliveries.

In Table above 43 ANC cases remained unaccounted for. It needs to be pointed out here that even if there has been one maternal death out of these it would mean a MMR of 286.5 and two deaths would make it a staggering 573 per 1,00,000 deliveries. The ANM's response to this anomaly was that there is in general a 10 per cent loss of cases between ANC registration and delivery. It is surprising that there should be a further loss of cases despite the ANM having already weeded out a substantial number of them by not registering women in the first trimester. Nevertheless, the argument of loss of cases can be conceded provided the probable reasons for the loss can be explained, which was not the case here.

With so much going wrong in practice, we naturally expect the staff to ensure that the possible adverse consequences of such practices are not reflected in the records. The observations made here may be accused of being based on a great deal of presumptive analysis. To impute motives where they do not exist is certainly not the idea here; however, based on the information that could be retrieved, we cannot but strike a note of caution. The question nevertheless remains that given these observations, to what extent can such an institutional delivery be considered a safe one; or is it that the blind drive to increase institutional deliveries imperilling the objective of safe deliveries which could well have been attempted by strengthening the traditional arrangements for maternal care?

In addition, poor nutrition is perhaps the single greatest cause of maternal morbidity and by implication mortality, but minimal effort seems to have gone into improving this aspect of maternal health in this drive to lower maternal mortality. It is important to note here that both the ANMs and the ASHA at Uleta sub-centre had practically no idea of what VHND (Village Health and Nutrition Day) is; neither has one been observed in the village over the past year, implying thereby that nutrition remains perhaps the most neglected aspect of maternal care.

The incentivization of deliveries has had another undesirable effect, i.e. the marginalization of the MPHW (M). As in rural areas the deliveries are conducted exclusively by females, especially in conservative areas like Mewat, the benefits of the incentives accrue only to the ANMs/MPHW(F). As the sub-centre focuses on RCH activities centred on women, with maximization of institutional deliveries forming the core of it, there is neither much work (except perhaps immunization) nor incentive for the MPHW(M) to be involved in the work of the sub-centre.

The motivation for performing institutional deliveries, overriding safety concerns, comes directly from the money to be made through incentives and non-formal payments. As is evident from Table, out of a total of 244 institutional deliveries, 217 were conducted at the sub-centre delivery hut. The incentive for the ANMs to perform deliveries comes after the first three deliveries of every month, and therefore the total number of non-incentive deliveries would be 72 per ANM at 3 non-incentive deliveries per month per ANM, there being two ANMs. Thus the ANMs received an incentive for performing the remaining 145 deliveries. Presuming the proportion of boys and girls to be equal at birth (in fact at birth the sex ratio is favourable to girls at 1,008 to 1,000) the total incentive on institutional deliveries works out to be Rs. 72,500 for the year 2010, i.e. Rs. 36,250 per ANM. This is a substantial amount and can be further enhanced by demanding non-formal payments from the relatives of the woman undergoing delivery. A survey of four women of Uleta village who had delivered over the past month at the sub-centre amply showed that non-formal payments were very much in vogue.

Besides, there is a definite possibility that many home deliveries are being shown as institutional ones to reap the rewards. This kind of occurrence was reported by some of the respondents in the households surveyed in the village as part of the study. One of the ANMs herself admitted that she had been performing deliveries at home if that was requested of her prior to the delivery hut at the sub-centre becoming operational. During the household survey, one of the respondents said that this particular ANM still performed deliveries at home and took money for the service. It however remains to be seen how long this spurt in the institutional deliveries at Uleta can be sustained in the absence of a genuine improvement in the standard of care.

It should be noted that only 6.2 per cent of the total number of women who gave birth at the centre benefited under the central JSY scheme while the beneficiaries of the state scheme was even fewer at just 2.3 per cent. This means that the actual benefits of the schemes to encourage institutional deliveries to the indigent pregnant women, who should have been the major beneficiaries, were very few, while the distortions that have crept into the practices due to monetary incentives have far outweighed the benefits.

It may also be noted that though both the ANMs at the sub-centre shared the same duties, the regular ANM earned twice the salary of the contract ANM. It was also observed by us that of the two ANMs, the one working on a contract basis was more active in performing deliveries. It should be no surprise then if the ANM working on a contract basis sees herself as disadvantaged and tries to make up for her perceived disadvantage by earning as much as she can through ethical/unethical institutional deliveries.

Therefore we see that at the level of the district health administration, improvement in the health status of Mewat was made synonymous with lowering maternal and infant mortality. Its practical implication was that in terms of service delivery the entire focus was the strategy of institutional deliveries and immunization. Further, at the level of the institution, as the focus was institutional delivery for which there were monetary incentives and for which answerability was sought, single-minded attention was devoted to institutional deliveries. The proportion of complete immunization was only 25 per cent and the quality of antenatal care, which is an integral and a key part of safe motherhood, was pitiable. Nothing could be a greater vulgarization of the concept of integrated preventive, promotive, and curative care than this narrowly focused techno-centric approach of boosting institutional deliveries. Even in this, the benchmarks are quantitative achievements and not qualitative outcomes.

This approach totally negates the role of the larger social determinants of health, cutting out the provision of health services from an integrated development strategy for the region. Let alone being aware of the social determinants of health, the health workers at the sub-centre were not even aware of the various strategies of the NRHM, of which institutional deliveries is only a part. Even though providing immunization and delivery facilities do cater to an aspect of the people's health needs, the overall functioning of the sub-centre fails to touch people's lives. Deliveries may take place at the most three or four times in a lifetime in a family for which it may look towards the sub-centre, but the need for curative care which may occur on a day-to-day basis remains unfulfilled. This cannot bode well for the public health services and their credibility with the the people. The result is that with respect to the daily lives of the people of Uleta village, the sub-centre stands in splendid isolation like a drop of oil in water.

Given the state of affairs as it stands there was scant evidence of intrinsic motivation either on the part of the health care providers to provide the health care services to the people for the sheer pleasure of it or on part of the people to actively participate in the functioning of the health centre and thereby to ensure the successful implementation of its services and to make it accountable to them because health services have an inherent value for their development. There was evidence to suggest that the value of extrinsic motivation in the form of monetary rewards for the health workers for institutional deliveries had been internalized by them as their own. Nothing could be more tragic for the cause of building a robust health system for the people of Uleta than this.

What Do We Surmise?

Relying on the foregoing discussion, we can hypothesize the following with regard to the implementation of health programmes:

- That the departure point for the implementation of health programmes should be faith in the people's innate ability to recognize their own welfare in optimally using health services and the willingness of the health workers to provide these services with the primary objective of contributing to society's welfare. The need is to provide conditions in which these innate abilities can gain maximum traction.
- That increasing commercialization of health care in India has provided 'social environmental influences' in which the provision of health services in return for pecuniary incentives has been internalized as a self-determined behaviour by many of the health workers instead of providing these services for their innate value for the development and well-being of the society.
- Commercialization of health care has led to a situation where the ability of the people to avail of health care, especially curative care, has become contingent upon their ability to pay for these services. Simultaneously, the quality of public sector health services leaves a great deal to be desired. Apart from this, people have a long experience of governments introducing health programmes in accordance with their own priorities rather than the people's need for easily accessible and affordable quality medical care. The massive family planning programme that was sought to be imposed through coercive means or extrinsic incentives is a notable example of this.
- This can be expected to lead to a lack of enthusiasm among the people for health services in the country. Therefore, their intrinsic motivation for the utilization of these services suffers. To overcome this invoking 'extrinsic motivation' of the consumers through monetary incentives appears to be the most convenient expedient for policy-makers to achieve public health goals.
- As against this, it is far more desirable that people and the

health workers jointly participate in the implementation of health programmes motivated by their inherent value. Therefore, compared to manipulation of people through 'extrinsic motivation' the governments and health administrators should seek to invoke the 'intrinsic motivation' of the people and the health workers for successful implementation of health programmes.

- That the psychological requirements of competence, autonomy, security, and relatedness to give full play to the intrinsic motivation of the people can best be fulfilled if health programmes are implemented as an integral part of the overall development strategy that takes in its sweep aspects like economic development, employment, housing, nutrition, education, public works, etc. in accordance with the fundamental objectives of Primary Health Care.
- More specifically, in consonance with the principles of Primary Health Care, the people should be involved at every step of the organization, operation, maintenance, and control of health services in order to leverage their intrinsic motivation to achieve public health goals through the implementation of health programmes.
- That such steps can be instituted only if the development paradigm, at least in the development sector, is freed from all commercial motives and the state ensures the availability of resources for running these services, including the resources required to fulfil the material needs of the health workers in consonance with the overall development of society.
- The policy-planners and administrators should use non-monetary social incentives for communities and also the health workers/providers to supplement their intrinsic motivation for successful implementation of health programmes. With regard to the health workers, their working conditions should be so designed as to maximally motivate them.

Conclusion

The greatest strides in the development of human civilization have been the result of mankind's collective aspiration to advance its well-being and a profound faith in its collective ability to foster the changes necessary for such advancement. Contrary to this, the market-led development paradigm posits consummation of individual human want/profit, as distinct from common societal good, as a necessary condition for the development of human society. This is most eloquently captured in the following words of one of the brashest proponents of the 'market', the former prime minister of the UK, Margaret Thatcher, who said: 'There is no such thing as society. There are individual men and women, and there are families. And no government can do anything except through people, and people must look after themselves first. It is our duty to look after ourselves and then to look after our neighbour' (Mackay Hugh, 2007). It is therefore not in the least surprising that the neoliberal model of development fails to recognize an 'innate human motivation' for achieving common good. For a market-driven development paradigm this is nothing but an unappetizing utopia.

Under the circumstances, providing individual incentives is presented as the best way forward to elicit people's participation in society's development. There is scarcely an example in history when people guided by their narrow self-interest have moved as a force to change the tide of events. There are of course innumerable examples when they were exhorted to rise above self, motivated by collective well-being and moved to change the course of human history. The question however remains of providing the conditions that will facilitate such a play of the human spirit.

China was an impoverished country with a huge burden of morbidity due to infectious diseases, mortality, hunger, poverty, and under-development when it set out on its journey to emerge as a modern nation in 1949. Its health services system existed only in name. Despite numerous experiments in development strategy, its fundamental policy approach to health emphasized 'preventive medicine and integrated development of health care with economic and social development'. Notwithstanding numerous challenges of a scarcity of resources and trained health manpower, during the

15 years between 1949 and 1965 smallpox, typhus, plague, and cholera were totally eliminated. Other diseases like tuberculosis, malaria, filariasis, schistosomiasis, trachoma, and ancylostomiasis, though still not fully controlled, were markedly reduced. These achievements were monumental considering the short span of a generation in which they were achieved. Though there was resistance to such efforts, as can only be expected in a class-divided society, efforts were made to encourage physicians and health workers to practise in rural areas. For example, in 1963, all medical students graduating from medical schools are said to have been assigned to the rural areas. Efforts such as raising an entire cadre of 'barefoot doctors' were actively supported by the state to mobilize the rural communities to take charge of their own health (Sidel and Sidel, 1982).

These achievements were possible not only through the logistical victory in provisioning the health services, but also due to the success in drawing on people's initiative in the organization of these services. The real development lies not as much in the physical infrastructure that is created, as in the liberating effect that such a creation has on the people. Without such a liberating effect, infrastructure could well be a source of misery. The following is an example of how industrialization was used to liberate women from orthodox oppression in the citadel of conservatism, Bokhara in the erstwhile Soviet Union, says it all. A girl textile worker of a silk mill in Bokhara wrote:

When I took the road to the factory
I found there a new kerchief,
A red kerchief, a silk kerchief,
Bought with my own hand's labour!
The roar of the factory is in me.
It gives me rhythm.
It gives me energy

(Strong, 1957)

In contrast, Thomas Hood's poem 'The Song of the Shirt' said this of Britain's factories in 1843:

With fingers weary and worn,
With eyelids heavy and red,

A woman sat, in unwomanly rags;
Plying her needle and thread.
Stitch, stitch, stitch, in poverty, hunger and dirt,
And still, with a voice of dolorous pitch,
She sang the song of the shirt

(Strong, 1957)

It is for the readers to judge the liberating experience that the implementation of Janani Suraksha Yojana can provide to the women of Mewat. In the meanwhile, it is our considered opinion that 'pay for performance' schemes are no alternative to the imperative of integrating the development of health services with the overall development of the society and to assure health workers that society will take care of all their needs in return for the services.

The readers might take respite in the fact that with the reports of malpractices by ANMs in the implementation of the Jachcha-Bachcha scheme piling up from different districts, the scheme now stands withdrawn; however, the implementation of JSY remains very much an incentive-driven scheme through much of the country and there remain serious issues with this strategy that need to be addressed.

REFERENCES

Anderson, R., S.T. Manoogian and J.S. Reznick (1976): The Undermining and Enhancing of Intrinsic Motivation in Preschool Children'. *Journal of Personality and Social Psychology*, vol. 34: 915–22.

Abduljawad, A., and A.F. Al-Assaf (2011): 'Incentives for Better Performance in Health care', *Sultan Qaboos University Medical Journal*, Vol. 11(2): 201-6.

Ashworth, M., P. Seed, D. Armstrong, et al. (2007): 'The Relationship Between Social Deprivation and the Quality of Primary Care: A National Survey Using Indicators from the UK. Quality and Outcomes Framework', *British Journal of General Practice*, Vol. 57: 441–8.

Ashraf, N., O. Bandiera, and K. Jack (2012): No Margin, No Mission? A Field Experiment on Incentives for pro-social tasks, Working Paper.

Amare, Y. (2011): Non-Financial Incentives for Voluntary Community health workers: A Qualitative Study, L10K Working Paper No. 2 (Addis Ababa: Ethiopia: The Last Ten Kilometres Project, JSI Research & Training Institute).

Bajpai, Vikas (2014): 'Implementation of the Janani Sishu Suraksha

Karyakram in Uttar Pradesh: Some Observations and Concerns', *Indian Journal of Social Work*, October 2014; Vol. 75 (4): pp. 573-594.

Basinga, P., P.J. Gertler, A. Binagwaho, et al. (2011): 'Effect on Maternal and Child Health Services in Rwanda of Payment to Primary Health-Care Providers for Performance: An Impact Evaluation.' *Lancet*, Vol. 377(9775): 1421–8.

Benabou, R. and J. Tirole (2003). 'Intrinsic and Extrinsic Motivation', *Review of Economic Studies*, Vol. 70 (3): 489-520.

Bhattacharyya, K., K. LeBan, P. Winch, M. Tien (2001): 'Community Health Worker Incentives and Disincentives: How They Affect Motivation, Retention, and Sustainability' (Washington DC: US Agency for International Development, Basic Support for Institutionalizing Child Survival Project (BASICS II)).

Covington, M.V., and K.J. Mueller (2001): 'Intrinsic versus Extrinsic Motivation: An Approach/Avoidance Reformulation, *Educational Psychology Review*, Vol. 13 (2): 157-76.

Csikszentmihalyi, M., and K. Rathunde (1993): 'The Measurement of Flow in Everyday Life: Towards a Theory of Emergent Motivation', in *Developmental Perspectives on Motivation* ed. J.E. Jacobs, (Lincoln: University of Nebraska Press), pp. 57-97.

Casalino, L., and A. Elster (2007): 'Will Pay-for-Performance and Quality Reporting Affect of (?) Health care Disparities?', *Health Affairs*, Vol. 26: w405-414.

Dongre, A. (2010): 'Effect of Monetary Incentives on Institutional Deliveries: Evidence from India', MPRA Paper No. 26339, August, available from http://mpra.ub.unimuenchen.de/26339/1/MPRA_paper_ 26339.pdf on January 23, 2014.

Deci, E.L., and R.M. Ryan (1985): *Intrinsic Motivation and Self-Determination in Human Behaviour* (New York: Plenum).

Deci, E.L. and R.M. Ryan (1991): 'A Motivational Approach to Self: Integration in Personality', in R. Dienstbier (ed.), Nebraska Symposium on Motivation, Vol. 38, Perspectives on Motivation (Lincoln: University of Nebraska Press), pp. 237-88.

deCharms, R. (1968): *Personal Causation*, (New York: Academic Press).

Deci, E.L. (1975): *Intrinsic Motivation*, New York: Plenum, quoted in Ryan and Deci, 2000b.

Deci, E.L., R. Koestner, and R.M. Ryan (1999): A Meta-Analytic Review of Experiments Examining the Effects of Extrinsic Rewards on Intrinsic Motivation. *Psychological Bulletin*, Vol. 125: 627-668.

Doran, T., E. Kontopantelis , J.M. Valderas et al. (2011): 'Effect of Financial Incentives on Incentivized and Non-Incentivized Clinical Activities: Longitudinal Analysis of Data from the UK. Quality and Outcomes

Framework', *British Medical Journal,* Vol. 342: d3590 doi: 10.1136/bmj.d3590.

Doran T., C. Fullwood , E. Kontopantelis, and D. Reeves (2008): 'Effect of Financial Incentives on Inequalities in the Delivery of Primary Clinical Care in England: Analysis of Clinical Activity Indicators for Quality and Outcomes Framework', *Lancet,* Vol. 372: 728-36.

Deci, E.L., R. Koestner, and R.M. Ryan (1999): 'A Meta-Analytic Review of Experiments Examining the Effects of Extrinsic Rewards on Intrinsic Motivation', *Psychological Bulletin,* Vol. 125 (6): 627.

Delhi State Report, District Level Household Survey 3 (New Delhi: Ministry of Health and Family and Mumbai: International Institute for Population Sciences).

Directorate of Economics and Statistics (2010): *Delhi Statistical Handbook* (NCR, Delhi: Government of Delhi).

Eisenberger, R., and J. Cameron, J. (1996): Detrimental Effects of Reward: Reality of Myth? *American Psychologist,* Vol. 51: 1153–66.

Ellingsen, T., and M. Johannesson M. (2008): 'Pride and prejudice: The Human Side of Incentive Theory', *American Economic Review,* Vol. 98 (3): 990–1008.

Fisher, C.D. (1978): 'The Effects of Personal Control, Competence, and Extrinsic Reward Systems on Intrinsic Motivation', *Organizational Behavior and Human Performance:* 21, 273–288.

Franco, L.M., S. Bennett, and R. Kanfer, (2002): 'Health Sector Reform and Public Sector Health Worker Motivation: A Conceptual Framework, *Social Science & Medicine*: 54(8), 1255–66.

Franco, L.M., S. Bennett, and R. Kanfer (2002): 'Health Sector Reform and Public Sector Health Worker Motivation: A Conceptual Framework', *Social Science & Medicine,* Vol. 54 (8): 1255–1266.

Government of India (GOI) (2007-8): 'District Level Household and Facility Survey under Reproductive and Child Health Project (DLHS-3), Fact Sheet Mewat, Ministry of Health and Family Welfare.

Gupta, S.K., Dinesh K. Pal, Rajesh Tiwari, et al. (2012): 'Impact of Janani Suraksha Yojana on Institutional Delivery Rate and Maternal Morbidity and Mortality: An Observational Study in India', *Journal of Health Population and Nutrition,* December, Vol. 30 (4): 464–71.

Golden, B.R. (2006): 'The Cost of Pay-for-Performance in Health care: An Alternative View', *Health Pap.,* Vol. 6(4): 39-46.

Gavagan, T.F., Du Hongya, B.G. Saver, et al. (2010): 'Effect of Financial Incentives on Improvement in Medical Quality Indicators for Primary Care', *Journal of American Board of Family Medicine,* Vol. 23 (5): 622– 31.

Gray, D.H.H. and J. Ciroma (1987): 'Attrition Among Village Health Workers in Rural Nigeria', *Socio-Economic Planning Sciences,* Vol. 22(1),

39-43.

Gertler P., and C. Vermeersch (2012): 'Using Performance Incentives to Improve Health Outcomes', World Bank Policy Research Working Paper No. 6100, Impact Evaluation Series No. 60 (Washington DC: The World Bank).

Gneezy, U., S. Meier, and P. Rey-Biel (2011): 'When and Why Incentives (Don't) Work to Modify Behaviour', *Journal of Economic Perspectives,* Vol. 25(4): 191-209.

Gneezy, U., and A. Rustichini (2000): 'Pay Enough or Don't Pay at All', *Quarterly Journal of Economics,* Vol. 115 (3): 791-810.

Hall, B.J., and J.B. Liebman, (1998): 'Are CEOS Really Paid Like Bureaucrats?', *Quarterly Journal of Economics,* Vol. 113(3): 653 – 91.

Johnson, F.A. (1993). *Dependency and Japanese Socialization* (New York: New York University Press).

Kesterton, A.J., John Cleland, Andy Sloggett, and Carine Ronsmans (2010): 'Institutional Delivery in Rural India: The Relative Importance of Accessibility and Economic Status', *BMC Pregnancy and Childbirth,* Vol. 10 (30).

Kamenica, E. (2012): 'Behavioural Economics and Psychology of Incentives', *Annual Review of Economics,* Vol. 4: 427-452.

Lazear, E.P. (2000): 'The Power of Incentives', *American Economic Review,* Vol. 90(2): 410–14.

Lindert, K. (2005): 'Bolsa Familia Programme: Scaling Up Cash Transfers for the Poor'. *MfDR Principles in Action: Sourcebook on Emerging Good Practices* (Washington D C: World Bank).

Lepper, M.R., Sheena Sethi, Dania Dialdin, and Michael Drake (1997): 'Intrinsic and Extrinsic Motivation: A Developmental Perspective', in *Developmental Psychopathology: Perspectives on Adjustment, Risk and Disorder',* ed. S.S. Luthar, J.A. Burack, D. Dicchetti, and J.R. Weiz (Cambridge) Cambridge University Press, 1997.

Miller, G., R. Luo, L. Zhang et al. (2012): 'Effectiveness of Provider Incentives for Anaemia Reduction in Rural China: A Cluster Randomized Trial', *British Medical Journal,* Vol. 345, e4809.

Miller, G., and K.S. Babiarz (2013): 'Pay for Performance Incentives in Low- and Middle Income Country Health Programmes', Working Paper 18932, National Bureau of Economic Research, Cambridge, USA.

McDonald, R., S. Harrison, K. Checkland, et al. (2007): 'Impact of Financial Incentives on Clinical Autonomy and Internal Mmotivation in Primary Care: Ethnographic Study', *British Medical Journal,* Vol. 334 (7608): 1357.

Maung, M., H. Kluge, T. Aye, et al. (2006): 'Private GPs Contribute to TB Control in Myanmar: Evaluation of a PPM Initiative in Mandalay

Division, *International Journal of Tuberculosis and Lung Disease*, Vol. 10 (9): 982-7.

National Institute of Health and Family Welfare (NIHFW) (2010): 'Evaluation of MAMTA Scheme in National Capital Territory of Delhi', Department of Planning and Evaluation, January, p. 3.

Oneindia News (2008): 'CM launches "Jacha Bacha Scheme" on I-day', August 15. Available from http://news.oneindia.in/2008/08/15/haryana-launches-jacha-bacha-scheme-on-i-day-1218792765.html on January 25, 2014.

Oxman, A.D., and A. Fretheim (2008): 'An Overview of Research on the Effects of Results-Based Financing', Report from Norwegian Knowledge Centre for the Health Services, *Systematic Reviews*, No. 16 –2008.

Phillips, J., F., W.L. Greene, and E.F. Jackson (1999): 'Lessons from Community-Based Distribution of Family Planning in Africa, Population Council Policy Research Division Working Paper No. 121 (New York, The Population Council).

Registrar General of India (RGI) (2009): *SRS Bulletin*, October, Vol. 44 (1): 1.

Registrar General of India (RGI) (2011): *Special Bulletin on Maternal Mortality in India 2007-09*, June.

Registrar General of India (RGI) and Centre for Global Health Research (CGHR), University of Toronto (2006): 'Maternal Mortality in India: 1997-2003; Trends, Causes and Risk Factors', Government of India, New Delhi.

Randive, B., V. Diwan, and Ayesha Da Costa (2013): 'India's Conditional Cash Transfer Programme (the JSY) to Promote Institutional Birth: Is There an Association between Institutional Birth Proportion and Maternal Mortality?' PLoS ONE 8(6): e67452. doi:10.1371/journal.pone.0067452.

Ryan, R.M., and E.L. Deci (2000a): 'Intrinsic and Extrinsic Motivations: Classic Definitions and New Directions', *Contemporary Educational Psychology*, Vol. 25: 54–67, doi:10.1006/ceps.1999.1020, available online at http://www.idealibrary.com.

Ryan, R.M. (1995). 'Psychological Needs and the Facilitation of Integrative Processes', *Journal of Personality*, 63, 397–427.

Ryan, R.M. and E.L. Deci (2000b): 'Self-Determination Theory and the Facilitation of Intrinsic Motivation, Social Development, and Well-Being', *American Psychologist*, Vol. 55(1): 68-78.

Ryan, R.M. (1995): Psychological Needs and the Facilitation of Integrative Processes, *Journal of Personality*, Vol. 63: 397–427.

Vallerand, R.J., and G. Reid (1984): 'On the Causal Effects of Perceived

Competence on Intrinsic Motivation: A Test of Cognitive Evaluation Theory', *Journal of Sport Psychology*: 6, 94–102.

Ryan, R.M. (1982), Control and Information in the Intrapersonal Sphere: An Extension of Cognitive Evaluation Theory', *Journal of Personality and Social Psychology*, 43, 450–61.

Ryan, R.M., and W.S. Grolnick (1986): Origins and Pawns in the Classroom: Self-report and Projective Assessments of Individual Differences in Children's Perceptions. *Journal of Personality and Social Psychology:* 50, 550–8.

Ryan, R.M., and J.G. La Guardia, (2000): 'What is Being Optimized Over Development?: A Self-determination Theory Perspective on Basic Psychological Needs Across the Life Span', in S. Qualls and R. Abeles (eds.), *Dialogues on Psychology and Aging* (Washington, DC: American Psychological Association Books).

Rosenthal, M.B., R. Fernandopulle, H.R. Song, and B. Landon (2004): 'Paying For Quality: Providers' Incentives for Quality Improvement', *Health Affairs*, 23(2): 127–41.

Ryan, A.M., and R.M. Werner (2013): 'Doubts About Pay-for-Performance in Health Care', *Harvard Business Review Blog Network*, October 9. Available from http://blogs.hbr.org/2013/10/doubts-about-pay-for-performance-in-health care/accessed on January 12, 2014.

Rusa, L., M. Schneidman , G. Fritsche et al. (2009): 'Rwanda: Performance-Based Financing in the Public Sector', in *Performance Incentives for Global Health: Potential and Pitfalls*, ed. R. Eichler and R. Levine (Washington DC: Centre for Global Development).

Regalia, F., and L. Castro (2009): 'Nicaragua: Combining Demand-and Supply-Side Incentives', in *Performance Incentives for Global Health: Potential and Pitfalls,* ed., R. Eichler and R. Levine (Washington DC: Centre for Global Development).

Singh, C.P. (2008): 'Feasibility Study of Mobile Medical Unit Operations in Mewat', Help Age India, Centre for Development of Corporate Citizenship, SP Jain Institute of Management and Research.

Sugathan, K.S., Vinod Mishra, and Robert D. Retherford (2001): 'Promoting Institutional Deliveries in Rural India: The Role of Antenatal-Care Services', National Family Health Survey Subject Reports, No. 20, International Institute for Population Sciences, Mumbai, India and East-West Centre, Population and Health Studies, Honolulu, Hawaii, US, December.

Singh, P. (2011): 'Performance Pay and Information: Reducing Child Malnutrition in Urban Slums', MPRA Working Paper.

Shen, Y. (2003): 'Selection Incentives in a Performance-Based Contracting System', *Health Services Research*, Vol. 38 (2): 535–52.

Sidel, R., and Victor W. Sidel (1982): *The Health of China* (London: Zed Books).

Strong, A.L. (1957): *The Stalin Era* (New York: Mainstream Publishers), p. 47.

The Institute of Rural Research and Development (IRRAD) (2006-7): 'Key Findings from the Baseline Report, Mewat and Kurukshetra', Available from http://www.smsfoundation.org/links/Baseline-Survey-Key-Findings.pdf and accessed on January 11, 2011.

Tonin, M., and M. Vlassopoulos (2012): 'Social Incentives Matter: Evidence from an Online Real Effort Experiment', Discussion Paper No. 6716, July, Institute for the Study of Labour, Bonn, Germany.

Victora, C., J. Vaughan, F. Barros, et al. (2000): 'Explaining Trends in Inequities: Evidence from Brazilian Child Health Studies', *Lancet*, Vol. 356: 1093–8.

World Health Organization (WHO) (1978): 'Report of the International Conference on Primary Health Care', Alma-Ata, USSR, September 6-12, 1978, Geneva.

Wilson, K.J. (2013): 'Pay-for-Performance in Health care: What Can We Learn from International Experience?', *Quality Management Health Care*, January-March, Vol. 22(1): 2-15. doi: 10.1097/QMH.0b013e31827dea50.

Wubneh, H.G. (1998): 'Child Survival Project and the Horses: An Alternative and Sustainable Approach to Child Survival Programmes', in *Presented Papers: High Impact PVO Child Survival Programmes*, Vol. 2, ed. B. Burkhalter and V. Graham, Proceedings of an Expert Consultation, Gaulladet University, Washington, DC, June 21-4.

World Bank (2004): 'World Bank Project Appraisal Document: Brazil Bolsa Familia Project, Report', No. 28544-BR, May 25, World Bank, Washington DC.

ANNEXURE

Table 1: Facility Survey of Sub-Centre Uleta for RCH Services

General Information	
Number of villages catered to by the sub-centre	6
Population covered by the sub-centre	9,362 (the norm is 5,000 per sub-centre)
Total no. of households under the sub-centre	1402
Population of Scheduled Caste households	478 in 105 households (5% of total population)
Total BPL (below poverty line) households	462 (33%)

Availability of Human Resources

Personnel	In Position	Vacant
ANM/Female health worker	One, at a salary of approx. Rs. 20,000 p.m.	-
Male health worker (MHW)	One (had not been reporting for duty for a long time and got himself transferred in January 2011. Currently there is one replacement MHW on a contract basis. Even the contract MHW was not present during our visits.	-
Additional ANM (contractual)	One (under RCH) at a consolidated salary of Rs. 10,000 p.m.	-
ASHA (accredited social health activist), a community health worker	5 as against the required strength of 9	There have never been more than five. In one village a a woman opted for ASHA training but withdrew when told that she is supposed to work voluntarily.
Sanitation staff	One sanitation worker has been informally engaged on a salary of Rs 400 per month which is spent from the untied fund.	There is no sanctioned post for a sanitation worker.
Immunization training	Yes	- Do -
Intra-uterine device (IUD) insertion training	Yes	- Do -
Integrated Management of Neonatal and Childhood Illnesses (IMNCI) training.	No	- Do -
Skilled birth attendant training.	Neither of the ANMs recalled any training other than their initial training in conducting deliveries.	- Do -

Physical Infrastructure

Water supply	
What is the main source of water supply?	There is no regular water supply; water has to be stored in cans.
Electricity	
Is power supply available?	Power supply is highly irregular, more regular in winter than in summer.
Toilet facility	
Is a functional toilet facility available?	There is one makeshift toilet that is used only by the sub-centre staff.
Delivery hut	
Does the sub-centre have a delivery hut?	Yes
Are the deliveries being conducted at the sub-centre?	Yes

Availability of Selected Furniture and Equipment*

Furniture	Available	Usable/Functional
Examination table	No	No
Labour table	Yes	Yes
Foot step	Yes	Yes
Cupboard with lock and key	Yes	Yes
Bedside screen	Yes	Yes
Instrument sterilizer	Yes	Yes
Auto-disposable (AD) syringes	Yes	-
Hub cutter B.P. Instrument**	NoYes	Not Functioning
Stethoscope	Yes	Functioning
Weighing machine (adult)	Yes	Yes
Weighing machine (for infants)	Yes	Functional
Haemoglobinometer	Yes	Not functional as reagents were not available
Foetoscope	Yes	No
SIMS speculum	Yes	Yes
IUD insertion kit	Yes	Yes
Vaccine Carrier	Yes	Yes

Drug Kits, Medicines, and Other Consumables Required for Control of Different Diseases

Item/Drug	Availability
Drug kit A: IFA tablets, ORS and Vit. A solution	Yes (all components)
Drug kit B: Tab. Methelergometrine Maleate 0.125mg, Inj. Methylergometrine (0.2mg/ml.), Tab Paracetamol (500mg), Tab.Mebendazole (100mg), Dicyclomine (10mg), Chloramphenicol eye ointment (250mg), Ointment Povidone Iodine (5%), Centrimide powder(125gm), absorbent cotton roll	Only Inj. Methylergometrine, Tab Paracetamol, Tab Mebendazole, Ointment Povidone Iodine and cotton rolls were available; but their supply is very irregular.
Testing strips for glucose in urine	Out of stock
Testing strips for proteins in urine	Not available

Services provided during the last month	
Number of haemoglobin estimation tests	None***
Number of urine test for presence of protein and sugar	Protein: None*** Sugar: None***
Number of deliveries conducted:	
· at home	None
· at sub-centre	27 (in Nov. 2010)
Number of post-natal care contacts made	No record available
Number of newborn care provided	No record available
Number of children treated for diarrhoea	None
Number of immunization sessions conducted	Immunization sessions are conducted on the 1st, 2nd, and 3rd Wednesday of the month in different villages. Besides this, special measles catch-up rounds were held in November and December 2010 in all the villages covered by the sub-centre.
Proportion of 100% immunized children	326 children out of approximately 1300 children under the age of five in the villages covered by the sub-centre, i.e. approximately 25%.
Number of school health check-ups organized	Never organized
Number of beneficiaries of Janani Suraksha Yojana (JSY) registered	None in November and December
Total money distributed and no. of beneficiaries under JSYCentral scheme under NRHM	Rs 12,300 to 19 beneficiaries (6.2% of total deliveries)
State government scheme for SCs	Rs 9,500 to 7 beneficiaries (2.3% of total deliveries)
Monitoring and Supervision Activities	
Have you prepared the sub-centre plan for this year?	The ANMs were unaware of the concept of an annual sub-centre plan, though they did mention monthly meetings of the VHSC (Village Health and Sanitation Committee) in which some decisions regarding the functioning of the sub-centre are taken along with discussion of other health issues concerning the village
When was the last sub-centre plan prepared?	Never prepared
Were you provided with any written feedback from the PHC?	No
During the last month has a medical officer visited the sub-centre?	Yes
During the last month has an LHV/ male health assistant visited the sub-centre?	A male health assistant (health inspector) visited in connection with the measles catch-up vaccination programme.
Do all the villages covered by your sub-centre have a Village Health and Sanitation Committee (VHSC)?	Only Uleta village has a VHSC

Has the VHSC been beneficial in the conduct of your activities?	Yes
Do you observe any Village Health & Nutrition Day (VHND)?	Not aware of VHND
Number of ASHAs identified in the villages covered by your sub-centre and received the first round of training?	There are 6 ASHAs and all have received the first round of training. One ASHA has been out of action for the past two months due to an injury. It is being proposed that even *dai*s (traditional birth attendants) be incorporated as ASHAs, even if illiterate, in order to make up the deficiency, but the proposal has yet to be cleared by the health administration.

*The ANMs said that they had asked for a suction machine to be provided to the centre, but this had not to date been provided.

**The LHV (lady health visitor) at the PHC, Nagina, said that the ANMs had not made a request for either the repair or the replacement of the BP instrument.

***No tests were being conducted at the sub-centre as the reagents had not been made available. When told this, the LHV (Lady Health Visitor) at the PHC, Nagina, who is supposed to supervise the work of the ANMs, said that the reagents are available but the ANMs have not placed a requisition for them. Nonetheless, as noted earlier, blood tests are not being conducted at the PHC either, and therefore this cannot be expected of the sub-centres.

Note: Though this information is important, for the sake of brevity, information on the physical condition of the sub-centre building, residential facilities for staff, training of the ANMs, waste disposal practices, and contraceptive supply for family planning have not been included here.

Index